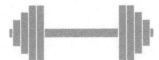

Stronger

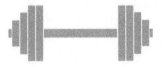

Stronger

How to build strength:
the secret to a
longer, healthier life

DAVID VAUX

First published in 2024 by Short Books
an imprint of Octopus Publishing Group Ltd
Carmelite House, 50 Victoria Embankment, London, EC4Y 0DZ
www.octopusbooks.co.uk

An Hachette UK Company
www.hachette.co.uk

10 9 8 7 6 5 4

A CIP catalogue record for this book is available from the British Library.

ISBN: 978-1-78072-609-0

Printed and bound in Great Britain by Clays Ltd, Elcograf S.p.A

This FSC® label means that materials used for the product have been responsibly sourced

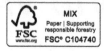

Cover design: Mel Four
Illustrations: Paul Palmer-Edwards
Typesetting and text design: Paul Palmer-Edwards
Cover text and design © Hachette UK Ltd

I wrote this book with the sole aim of democratising strength training. I have attempted to walk the middle ground by sharing effective, friendly, reliable and hopefully entertaining information. The process was informed by the strength journeys of the inspirational individuals I have worked with, as well as my own observations and research into how to win at ageing.

To this end, I urge you to read this book as it has been written, from beginning to end. That way, you will learn the important lesson of 'why' before tackling the 'what', and will be far more likely to commit to a lifelong journey towards a stronger, independent future.

CONTENTS

Introduction

One of my most valuable life lessons was given to me by a patient with whom I worked in the last five years of her life. Joy was tall, lean and full of energy, with a fierceness of spirit that shone out of her eyes. She was interested in everything and everyone.

'I have been dancing all my life and need you to help me continue' were her first words to me. She was 88 and I had never heard a cooler opener!

Over the next five years as Joy's osteopath, I would see her every six weeks to help with pain or mobility issues and give suggestions on strength-maintaining activity. Joy would bring me books and recommend podcasts and films. She never failed to teach me something. She was still interested in life, making new friends and learning until the day she died aged 93. Joy passed away peacefully in her own bed, with no illness, no medication or need for care, whilst living the life that she wanted. I have no doubt she had interesting plans for the very day that turned out to be her last. Being active until she died was hard evidence of what I had studied and continue to observe in my work on healthy ageing:

Strength is the magic bullet for a full, enjoyable and independent life right up to our last day on this planet.

Joy had a genetic pedigree of family longevity, a little luck, a positive mindset and commitment to lifelong regular exercise and learning. However, first and foremost Joy had built and maintained the neuromuscular system that literally propelled her through the day and kept her immune system working well. She was a strong woman in every sense and showed me that vitality and power is possible for everyone, no matter what age they start strengthening.

As an osteopath, I have worked to help individuals with pain and arthritis, and international sports teams with conditioning and medical advice. I have also worked on UK public health projects, and with think tanks on wellbeing in ageing. For many years, I served as a fire service physical education officer and I am a lifelong fitness enthusiast. My personal motivation to maintain strength has come from my lived experience following an injury that ended my career as a firefighter, when it proved an effective part of my recovery, and my own journey into middle age.

As I was to find after the injury that changed my life, recovery is not always a case of surgery, rehab and then return to work. The mental fall-out of losing my identity, so wrapped up within my firefighter's uniform, proved to be as persistent as the back and leg pain that still lingers today. It would take five years before I was able to manage my pain to the point that I did not need medication. What I discovered was that prolonged exposure to pain was not only draining me physically but also damaging every aspect of my life.

Although it is frustrating to be told that pain is 'all in your head' when you feel it very acutely in your body, to a certain extent it is true. Pain lives in our brains along with our consciousness; a bit like a nuisance neighbour who you wish would move away. When pain affects our strength and ability to move, this nuisance neighbour becomes louder and more annoying until they drown out all other thoughts.

It was my injury that changed my entire outlook on strength, movement and exercise. Far from being merely an element of physical performance, I found that as I slowly regained my strength, my pain changed for the better. I was much less aware of that annoying neighbour. I realised that having strength was just as intrinsic to my wellbeing as eating or breathing.

What I learned transformed how I help people invest in their future health and now I want to pass that knowledge on to you, so that you can secure yours. I had become an expert in older-age strength only to realise that middle age (for our purposes, the years between 35 and 65), was in fact the key period to influence it meaningfully. However, I also understood that I was in the minority, because very few people have any idea that strength training is the single most important factor affecting older-age health. Fewer still realise that middle age is a key life stage in which the quality of our future health can be determined.

Joy, alongside many others I have seen flourish in older age, had built up her strength before and into middle age. With my support she had continued to do this until the day she died. During our sessions, I would suggest an everyday activity that would keep her legs strong or help with balance, such as holding a static squat position when in her 'little room'. We would laugh at this, but it was a reminder that leg strength work can be done anywhere, at any time – even if it happens to be in the smallest room in the house!

Can you stand up from sitting in a deep or low chair without using your hands?

- Can you stand on one leg whilst putting a sock on the other foot?
- Do you find it easy to climb over stiles or fences if out walking?
- Do you find it easy walking down staircases or steps?

If you have answered no to any of the questions above, you should consider improving your thigh and hip strength. If you answered yes to all the questions – great! Let's learn how to keep things this way!

Keeping stronger for longer

So why is strength so important? Well, I am not alone in believing that the *stronger* we are, the *longer* we live with our independence and health intact. A decade-long observational study found those with the lowest muscle mass and strength levels had around double the mortality risk compared to the control group. Not surprisingly, they also found that those with low strength and muscle mass, plus a combination of diabetes, high blood pressure and obesity, were found to have over three times the risk of mortality.[1] I believe that by consistently working on our long-term muscle mass and strength, whilst maintaining healthy weight, we are highly likely to enjoy better quality of life and health in old age. If we also have good cardiovascular fitness, then the odds of enjoying versus enduring our older age are going to keep increasing.

The decline in muscle and strength due to ageing has been a preoccupation of humans since early Greeks and Romans first wrote despairingly about the loss of youthful vigour.[2] In the 20th century, the term 'sarcopenia' (from the Greek 'sarx' or flesh, and 'penia' or loss) was coined to denote this decline and the associated frailty it causes.

Simply put, being frail means we lack the reserves to recover from illness, injury or other life events that would normally not impact our health. Frailty makes us more vulnerable to falls, fractures and physical decline, often leading to admission to care settings and even premature death.

The good news is that frailty can be improved by prioritising the preservation of skeletal muscle strength for older age. But before we relax, thinking we can delay getting stronger until some future time, be warned – if we leave it too late, we could miss our chance. It is during middle age that we still have a window of responsiveness to exercise that can help to significantly improve our long-term muscle mass, strength and power. Furthermore, it is in middle age that adaptations leading to sarcopenia and frailty start, subtly at first and then more noticeably. It is true that we can build some strength in our sixties, seventies and even eighties, but it'll be much harder and for some, impossible. When discussing this subject with Rachel Copper, professor of epidemiology within the age research group at the University of Newcastle, she suggested a *cumulative* beneficial effect from long-term strength training. Similar to a pension plan, it seems the sooner in life we start strength training, the better!

There are some factors affecting our strength that we can't change. All humans experience hormonal decline, typically starting in our mid-thirties, that we can do little to influence. But we also lose strength in middle age due to general inactivity, ineffective strength training or through focusing too heavily on non-strengthening exercises.

It is these last three factors that are our focus, because that's what we can control. If we engage in strength training at the right time in our lives, we can transform our future health. We will be much less likely to become frail, need care, get injured or die before our time due to illness or as a consequence of falling.

Why now?

If you are reading these words and feel that this does not apply to you because you are 30 or 40, or because you are exercising regularly, it's time to think again. In my experience, most of us feel that this information is irrelevant to us. Who cares about what happens in 30 years' time? This mindset is understandable, and I certainly was guilty of it myself, especially as I was a regular participant in a broad spectrum of activities such as running, swimming, cycling and hiking. I thought I had exercise covered, and certainly hadn't considered my own mortality! However, what I was seeing in my clinic and in my research told a different story. I realised I was as much at risk of later-life frailty as anyone else.

Many of us may have gone to a gym in our late teens and twenties to build muscle and strength. But the number of people in their forties, fifties or sixties doing the same make up a small percentage of the population. Equally worrying is the fact that most people, of any age, don't know and haven't been educated about strength. Think about it: what do you most associate with strength training? Younger people in expensive-looking sports gear? Perhaps uninviting gyms, awash with protein shakes and loud music? Worse still, sweaty muscle-bound types taking selfies to post later? Social media and advertising have perhaps helped to reinforce the myth that strength training is the preserve of the young. But this is simply not true, and my mission is to bust this myth, and democratise strength for one and all.

In the past I have worked on steering groups focused on initiatives to get older people and those in care homes to be more active. I have seen the positive effects that engaging and supporting older age groups or those with long-term conditions can have. However, research and my own experience in clinic suggest that older age is not the best time to start building strength. Unfortunately, if an older person stops following the strength advice they were given, any improvements will be very short-lived. Moreover, short-term exercise interventions can do more harm than good. It seems obvious to me that anything achieved quickly in terms of building strength can be lost just as swiftly. The same pattern is seen with rapid weight loss and crash dieting. It is far better to allow your body to become stronger over the long term if that strength is to be maintained. One of the UK's leading campaigners for optimal health in older age, Professor Sir Muir Grey, is on the same page. He argues that major health problems from biological ageing do not appear until the age of 90 or older, and many signs that are commonly attributed to ageing, such as weakness, stiffness, shortness of breath and fatigue, are in fact due to loss of fitness. I wholeheartedly agree. The best prescription for staying young is to make an early investment in your strength and fitness, taking little steps every day to delay the signs of ageing for as long as possible.

We need to give ourselves the time to become fluent in strength, which, like learning a language, can take years. But once we have it mastered, it will literally act as a font of youth, or more aptly, a reservoir.

Your strength reservoir

Think of your personal strength as a beautiful mountain reservoir. If the reservoir is full, it has the capacity to feed your needs: to move, to maintain good posture, to avoid trips and falls, and underwrite your immune system. This is a useful metaphor since our skeletal muscle also acts as a real physical reservoir of amino acids, stored within our muscle proteins. There are 20 types of amino acids, nine of which we get from our food. Proteins are made up of chains of amino acids that come together to execute the individual task in hand. At an everyday level, it is our amino acids that allow our bodies to conduct their housekeeping duties. These include the growth and repair of muscle and other body tissues, including tendons and ligaments, the making of antibodies, hormones and enzymes that are essential for human life and the maintenance of healthy skin, nails and hair. The reservoir of amino acids contained within our skeletal muscle can also be drawn on as an energy source.

As we age, the level of the reservoir will naturally begin to drop, but can be topped up via our exercise and lifestyle choices, which will prevent us from becoming frail.

By keeping our reservoir topped up via strength training, we are more likely to be able to respond to whatever life throws at us – whether that be illness, accident or unforeseen immobility due to surgery. It will help us maintain our ability to move and in turn increase the likelihood of living independently in older age.

Something as simple as the ability to perform an own body weight squat is one of the main predictors of whether we will need care in later life. A squat is the main movement required to get on and off the toilet independently, the ability to get in and out of bed or navigate a staircase. What seem like everyday activities to most of us might one day take on life-changing significance. So it's a good idea to occasionally test yourself in this movement either on a chair, or anything else you tend to sit on every day!

Bonus feature: maintaining strength in this movement will also protect our bones, making them less likely to fracture in an accident. It also reduces the chances of falling as our balance will benefit.

Lower-body strength check

Are you sitting comfortably? Then let's begin with a lower-body strength check.

- From your seated position and without using your arms, try standing up using only your thigh muscles.
- If this is too easy, make it harder by trying the same movement from a lower chair.
- You can further challenge yourself by trying to stand up using only one thigh, and then lastly standing up from a seated position on the floor (again, without using your arms).
- If the chair test is not possible for you without the aid of your arms, you can make things easier by adding cushions to the seat of your chair until you can progress to the examples above as you become stronger.
- For every version of this movement, try standing and then slowing the lowering phase for the count of 4 seconds. This lowering under control is called an *eccentric* contraction and is gold dust for older-age strength. We will be discussing this and what other types of muscle contractions can offer later in the book.

Strength vs exercise

Let's face it, we've all been guilty of avoiding exercise at some point. Perhaps we've had an exhausting week or it just doesn't fit into a busy schedule. That said, you might still be surprised to hear that in the UK we spend more time on the toilet than engaged in exercise.[3]

When we dig deeper, we see that those who *are* participating in exercise tend to focus on aerobic-type activity such as swimming, cycling or running. Historically this was, and continues to be, driven by fitness messages focused on getting outside and 'getting a sweat on'. This has great merit in terms of burning calories, maintaining healthy weight and preventing diabetes and heart disease. But despite the benefits, aerobic-type activity is not enough to offer maximal protection from things like frailty and osteoporosis in older age – unless it is combined with the magic ingredient: regular strength training.

I believe that an overemphasis on aerobic-type activity has had a negative consequence on the strength levels of nations around the world. It has led to what I refer to as 'strength hesitancy', which was confirmed by a recent survey in the UK that found that only 7% of men and 4% of women achieved the recommendations for strengthening activity.[4] This in spite of the fact that the National Health Service and the World Health Organization both recommend that adults strength train all major muscle groups twice a week.[5] The lack of strength across an individual's entire life can have devastating effects not only on their quality of life in older age, but also the wider community who support them.

The trick is maintaining a balance between the two. We need to value cardiovascular *and* strength training, and devise a way to incorporate both into our exercise plans. The last thing we want is for people to pivot to only strength training and create a new 'sweat hesitancy'. We need to get a sweat on AND build our strength up!

Don't stop moving

My epiphany in my own strength journey came from learning that the key to staying strong is never to give up.

I am sure we can all think of people, family or colleagues perhaps, who were once known for being fit, strong and capable. Perhaps as a young person we aspired to be as accomplished as them one day. Such a moment came for me when, at the age of 18, I first met my recruit fire instructor station officer. He was a no-nonsense officer who had seen and done it all in the fire service. He was able to bench press 300 pounds and run a marathon in under three hours. But his party trick was to climb, hand over hand, up a 30-foot fireman's pole using only his upper body and with his legs held at a right angle. He was 45 years old at the time.

For many years, I believed that, like my recruit station officer, being fit and strong at one point in my life would protect me in older age. I was in fact buying into one of the most common exercise myths. I have since learned that former physical fitness is no guarantee of a healthy or pain-free older age. This even applies to former professional athletes; they are not protected from frailty or ill health in later life unless they continue with a healthy lifestyle which includes regular strength training.

As we will explore later, there are many examples of strong, powerful individuals who prove that being athletic at the age of 80 is an achievable goal for any of us. The secret is to never stop trying. We can't afford to rely on former glories or past behaviours. We can, however, rely on good foundations and habits that we have built. Our past actions are the past. We really are only as good as our last exercise session or meal. Historic levels of fitness or strength are only relevant if we have continued to build on them without long periods of inactivity.

The exercise and lifestyle choices we commit to in middle age will preserve our strength and health into older age.[6,7] I like to think of a long-term commitment to strength training as similar to welcoming a lifelong companion into my life. A companion that helps to support and inspire me to reach a stronger, safer older age. Just like those firm but encouraging instructions my recruit station officer barked, some 32 years ago, when I was on the brink of physical exhaustion during a heat and humidity exercise: 'Don't you stop now, Vaux!'. I fully intend not to.

Health span vs strength span

Imagine strength as your physical pension; the sooner you start to build and maintain it, the better and more rewarding your older age will be. Just as financial planning is important for a happy retirement, so too is physical planning.

Fortunately, much can be done to maximise our chances of better strength in our older years if we engage with the 'strength-span' approach in middle age (or earlier). Health-span is a term we use to describe the concept of living longer whilst enjoying robust health levels and independence. But strength-span is even more important than this – it is a lifestyle and exercise approach that underpins our ability to achieve health-span. It prioritises our health and strength during middle age onwards.

Unfortunately, it is this very time in life that often seems to be the busiest, with many of us juggling stressful jobs and multiple responsibilities, including caring for children and/or parents. It is the middle-aged who have the most to gain and lose during this already hectic period. It can also be a very vulnerable time in terms of losing sight of our later life health and starting to notice the ageing process, with women also having to contend with the menopause. Thankfully, there are simple actions we can take to set our compass towards a healthy older age. Middle age is the time to change the narrative and normalise strength training. This book will help you do just that.

A 10-second test

Can you stand on one leg for more than 10 seconds with little or no trouble?

As well as improving balance, the act of standing on one leg will strengthen your core and hip muscles on both sides, whilst also improving leg strength and foot stability on the standing leg. Try it both sides to see if there is a difference. If you can go longer than 10 seconds, great work! Now try to get to a minute – and do this whilst brushing your teeth for extra credit.

You probably did this as a child without a second's thought. If you are in your twenties or thirties, maybe you can still do it without too much trouble. But if you are in your forties or fifties, is it still as easy? The chances are that if you have remained active and exercised you can probably complete it, but perhaps not as easily as before? Frustratingly, it isn't going to get any easier when you get older unless you start building your balance, strength and power now. In fact, it is probably going to get a good deal harder.

Why is this so important? Well, the ability to maintain your balance can potentially save you from a life-changing fall. It is the interactions and postural corrections we make within the nervous system and the skeletal muscle that keep us balanced.[8] Stronger muscles provide better information to our brains to achieve this balance. If you often find yourself wobbling and falling, then larger, faster muscle contractions may be needed to keep you upright. Therefore, the ability to rapidly contract a muscle has a significant role to play in preventing stumbles.

The important message to remember here is that maintaining regular strength training can improve the relationship between our nervous system and muscles (more on this later). This mind–body relationship works to improve balance and reduce the likelihood of falling and injury in older age.

Clearly, the relationship between our nervous and muscular systems contains helpful mechanisms that remain dormant in many of us due to inactivity. With this in mind, simple balance exercises that engage the nervous system, and regular body-wide strength training with emphasis on quick contraction of muscles, should be considered as important as healthy weight, cholesterol and cardiovascular fitness.

Living longer and better with strength

I want to encourage you to see strength as the foundation to all other exercise or healthy lifestyle choices. Given the generally upward trend in life expectancy, if you are currently middle-aged, you stand a good chance of living into your eighties or even nineties.[9] With advances in modern screening and medicine, longevity will no doubt continue to creep up.

During my time in fire rescue, we lived by the ethos of training hard to protect you from your 'worst day'. We strived to be as proficient with our equipment and as physically ready as was humanly possible. This was for a simple reason: being as strong as we could be might, on that 'worst day', save your life and ours. In a different way, this book is here to help protect you on your own worst day!

Personally, I believe our worst day to be the day when we literally run out of the strength required to walk, stand, climb stairs or just live independently and do the activities we enjoy. We all have it within our control to make sure that this does not happen prematurely, or indeed at all for some of us.

I'm rooting for you

The pursuit to maximise later-life strength should be a national obsession. Many of us seem to believe that being an athletic and strong older person is the preserve of the lucky few who have the genetics, wealth, education or lifestyle to achieve it. Far from it.

In taking a dive into strength, you will discover why this subject has personal, national and global importance. You will explore new scientific breakthroughs on how to age well via lifestyle and strength activity, whilst dismissing less useful and sometimes harmful claims from the fitness industry. If you are not exercising at all, or not doing much, this book will help you get motivated to start doing the right kinds of exercise now. If you feel you are exercising well already, I hope you'll find something new here. You might even discover what you thought you knew about exercise was in fact a myth. You might find you are overtraining, or focusing on the wrong exercises – and by making subtle changes, be able to significantly improve your health and long-term resilience.

I've written this book using words that the older me will be grateful to have heard, and that I wish my parents had received in their middle age. In the coming chapters, we will explore the natural miracle that is our neuromuscular system, and how we can better utilise all of it to our advantage. We will explore different ways to think about strength, discovering how to achieve it and, most importantly, hold onto it once we have it. I will reveal what I have learned within my own and my patients' journeys in and out of injury and pain by harnessing innate mechanisms that for many remain unused. We will discuss protein, the importance of recuperation and how to prepare for strength training, and then explore which 10 movements will help us build strength to *finish the race strongly* within the coming chapters. I'll start by exploring the biological systems in our bodies and how to keep them healthy, so that you are fully equipped with the most practical tools for understanding how to maintain strength across your entire life.

My message is simple – no one has as much influence on your later-life health, independence and happiness as you yourself do. Becoming stronger is a journey we all need to make. As with any other journey, looking at a map will help start us on the best path.

Part 1

1

The Strength Map of the Body

'A chain is no stronger than its weakest link.'
Thomas Reid, 1786

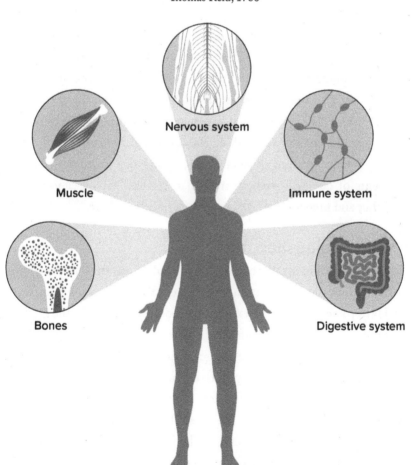

We are all familiar with young men who obsess over the size of their biceps or 'guns'. I was one of them 35 years ago, focused only on trying to get my own *guns* and other muscles as big as possible. I had no concept of what other biological systems were involved in this process until years later, when I started taking my training seriously as a competitive rower and operational firefighter. Even then, however, I was all about the performance side of training, and it was only when I started to train as an osteopath that I was able to navigate my way out of injury and pain. This was because I learned about the many incredible processes and systems in the body that are required to build strength and keep it up. In the same way, I want to show you how becoming stronger and building a body fit for old age is not just about isolated muscle groups but a *networked* process.

The systems required to make and keep us strong involve many complex biological interactions: think of them as an orchestra, made up of many sections such as brass, string, percussion and woodwind. By themselves, these sections are important and have huge potential, but when combined in concert, they produce something truly powerful. Similarly, our muscles, bones, nervous system, connective tissues and digestive system are all elements of our own strength map that we need to consciously bring together and tune for our best chance of a healthy old age.

Diet and digestion

First, let's explore an often-overlooked tool in our muscle-preserving armoury: our digestive system – the system that feeds our muscles.

Have you ever heard the expressions 'bodies are made in the kitchen, not the gym', or 'you can't outrun a bad diet'? There's an important truth behind these sayings. Before we get into exploring the strength map and understanding those key muscles in more detail, it's essential to understand the vital role nutrition plays: it is the one of the most important factors affecting the loss of muscle as we age. Just as important as strength training itself, having a sufficient intake of proteins is key to building and maintaining our muscle mass. Strength training without paying attention to protein intake is like servicing your car but using the wrong type of fuel. Proteins and their building blocks, amino acids, have many vital biological functions, including building and maintaining our skeletal muscle. As you are probably aware, a multi-billion-dollar industry in protein supplements has grown up in recent years. I am an advocate of any form of protein as part of a healthy diet, be it from food or ethically approved supplements. Whichever way you choose to get your proteins is down to your own personal budget, ethical standpoint and the time you have to invest in it. Just make sure that you are getting the correct amount and the best quality possible, because otherwise, your entire biological system could be compromised in the long run, not just your muscle strength.

One of the challenges we all face is that as we age, our ability to absorb proteins significantly decreases.[1] Let's imagine that we have a green light in our heads that indicates that if we are efficiently absorbing the protein from a meal or supplement after exercising. In a person in their twenties or thirties, the light can stay on for many hours, sometimes over twelve. This number reduces to just a few hours in a person in their forties or fifties, and perhaps just an hour in a person aged 75. In fact, there have been many studies that suggest the older we get our systems instead *resist* the absorption of proteins. This is yet another explanation for why older relatives might seem painfully thin or frail. Not only did they not built up enough muscle in middle age, but now, in older age, they are disadvantaged in maintaining what little muscle they have.

All is not lost though, because if we are strength-training in mid life (or at any age for that matter), it increases our levels of protein absorption, helping our green light stay on for longer.[2] If an older person does not do strength-based exercise, protein supplements will not be as effective – it would be like putting the right fuel into a car that has not been carefully serviced and whose bodywork is beyond repair. There are many theories that advocate different methods of maximising protein absorption – choosing a particular time of day to eat protein or aligning *this meal* with *that work out* to optimise uptake. Although there does seem to be some logic to such eating strategies, I am also mindful that the average middle-aged person will not have the time or capacity to put all this in place. If you are new to strength training, I would instead just make sure you are getting enough protein, whether through meat, dairy or vegan and vegetarian products. Needless to say, it's not merely the amount, but also the quality of the proteins we ingest that is important to building strength.

As a rule of thumb, a middle-aged person who is strength-training should aim to have around 1.2–1.5g of proteins per kg of their body weight. This means a 100kg person needs 120–150g a day. In conversations with Martin Lau, one of the UK's leading dieticians (with a special interest in seniors' fitness), he pointed out that there is an emerging pattern of research that advocates 'eating protein at every meal'. For example, around 30g of protein three or four times a day, which can also include snacks between meals, such as nuts, protein drinks or other options, such as boiled eggs. This certainly make sense, given that we want to be ready with proteins in our system, whatever time our 'green light' comes on. If in doubt, I always advise opting for a little more protein, particularly if you feel you are not progressing after a few months of strength training.

As we will touch on later in this chapter, our body composition and excess fat tissue have a direct impact on our long-term health and ability to maintain our skeletal muscle mass. There is now a great deal of research to suggest that adopting a Mediterranean-style diet and watching portion size is an effective long-term lifestyle change that can help maintain our weight and indeed health deep into older age.[3]

All-day protein-rich foods

Breakfast
Greek yogurt and kefir
Milk and other dairy
Eggs
Nut butters, eg. peanut, almond and cashew

Lunch and dinner
Lean meat and poultry
Seafood
Legumes such as beans, lentils, chickpeas and soybeans

On the go
Unprocessed nuts and seeds

Muscling in

Now we've understood the important role of nutrition and protein in helping us build strength, let's take a closer look at strength itself, and perhaps most crucially: muscle. Muscle appears in three forms. The first type is smooth muscle, which is found within many organs of the body, including those in the digestive or reproductive systems, and also lines blood vessels. The second is cardiac muscle, which is found in the walls of the heart and contracts to pump blood around the body. Both smooth and cardiac muscles function automatically until the day we die. In relation to our cardiac muscle, it is without doubt essential to include regular aerobic and some anaerobic (more intense) exercise in our lives to keep the heart in good condition, maintain efficiency in different energy systems and help with managing healthy weight (more on this later).

It seems obvious to state, but the quality of any cardiovascular workout is only as good as the strength of our skeletal muscles to perform. Which brings us to the third form, skeletal muscle, which is attached to our bones via tendons and is the only type of muscle that is under our voluntary control, meaning we must consciously command it to move. It is the strength of our skeletal muscle that forms the foundation on which all other health-related or everyday activities rely. In fact, greater muscle mass is associated with attaining higher levels of 'maximal aerobic capacity', or VO_2 max – the maximum amount of oxygen our bodies can consume during high-intensity exercise.[4] The fact that having strong muscles increases our aerobic capacity shows that it's possible to train for both strength and aerobic fitness at the same time. However, if you want to go for a run or walk, you first need to have the required strength to get up from your chair! Skeletal muscle is second only to the brain in its metabolic activity, so the more skeletal muscle we have, the greater the calories burnt during exercise and at rest, which can be helpful in our efforts to maintain heathy body weight and prevent type 2 diabetes.

Skeletal muscle

Our skeletal muscles account for around 40% of our total body weight. This percentage can vary across individuals, with women tending to have a little less muscle in their upper body than men. We can expect the voluntary loss of muscle mass to start in our thirties, from which point the rate of loss is 3–8% per decade.[5] As we reach our sixth decade, this rate becomes even higher. Sadly, this is often seen in our elderly relatives, who seem to be slowing down for a prolonged period and then suddenly age very quickly.

Let's stop and consider this fact for a moment. If we live 30–40 years after middle age, that's a significant loss of skeletal muscle mass. By the time we reach 80, it's possible that some of us may have lost around 30% of our skeletal muscle mass and in particular the fast-twitch muscle fibres, which we will explore in this chapter.

A good tailor will ensure that your outfit has seams that are strong in every direction and select the best material. Likewise, operational firefighting gear is reinforced in areas more prone to wearing out and made from fire-resistant fabric. In the sections below, I will explain the different areas in the body and why they need to be strengthened so that we can construct our very own 'age-resistant suits'. But before that, let's take a look at how we can acquire the best material for the job in hand.

Slow- and fast-twitch fibres: the stronger fabric

We have three main types of skeletal muscle fibres: slow twitch and two types of fast twitch. For the purpose of this book, we will refer to them as 'slow-twitch', 'fast-twitch' and 'difficult-to-reach' fibres (a subset of the fast-twitch type). Everyday tasks that are relatively easy to perform are more dependent on slow-twitch fibres, whilst moderate to hard activity that requires increased speed and strength, we use our fast-twitch and difficult-to-reach types. Fast-twitch fibres are intrinsic to building strength across the human body. Now let's take a look at the different regions, where we need to build strength in our skeletal muscle:

Upper body

If we think of our skeleton as a fortress, and we should, no fortress is going to last long if we only have defences on one or two sides. In other words, we need to be strong in all the major directions of movement to protect our bones and joints from injury.

Upper-body strength is essential in allowing us to engage with the environment around us via our hands. To do so, we need to be strong in our shoulders, chest, back and arm muscles. It's all very well being able to do a press-up (a horizontal push); however, if in your old age you had to lift a heavy case into an overhead locker (a vertical push), you would be very likely to get injured had you not trained for this movement in prior decades. Similarly, you may be great at lifting things into overhead lockers if you have trained that muscle group, but if you have neglected to work on vertical pulls, you are heading for trouble in your latter years if you need to pull yourself up after a fall.

Lower body

Given that the largest area of muscle of the body is in our legs, we need to keep them strong to ensure we avoid frailty and maintain our ability to move well – the ability to climb stairs, stand, walk, use the bathroom or just get from A to B are all reliant on the strength required to perform a lunge or squat. It will be harder to retain the strength in our lower limbs in later life, so we need to be diligent in middle age to gain a good level of strength and power in this area, and then work to hang onto as much of it as we can for the rest of our lives. We can all benefit from building stable, powerful and athletic legs that will literally carry us through our older age, efficiently and safely.

Hips

Think of standing up straight or bending down to pick something up from the ground, and you will have imagined a classic hinging movement that is driven by the strength of the muscles surrounding our hips, including the largest muscles in our bodies – our bum (gluteal muscles) and the back of our thighs (hamstrings). Being strong in this hinging movement improves our gait and standing posture whilst also toning and strengthening the glutes. Much of our older-age physical ability relies on this movement, which is why it joins the lunge and squat as an essential strength exercise to propel us into a healthy older age.

Core

The core is the midsection of the body and includes the interaction between the abdominal (stomach) muscles and lower back. Strength in this region influences all human movement, acting as a bridge between our upper and lower bodies and also braces our lower back. It protects us from back injury and underpins our posture in older age. Becoming stronger in our core not only allows us to lift and carry things but also provides a body-wide strengthening effect.

Grip

A strong grip is driven by good muscle strength in our forearm and the intrinsic small muscles of the hand, and is central to older-age health, happiness and wellbeing. In many ways, it can come to define our independence, acting to protect us in everyday life. Our ability to use our hands not only helps us in daily tasks like opening jars, cooking, carrying shopping or holding cups and plates but can also increase the chances of saving ourselves from a fall, by grabbing onto something when we trip. In older age, our ability to save ourselves from falling can have profound consequences. Improving grip strength has also been shown to enable a body-wide strengthening effect.

The nervous system as the conductor

Building a strong musculoskeletal frame is not just about muscle. There are other key systems we should be aware of when working towards a stronger older age. Going back to my earlier analogy, if the muscle, bone and connective tissue make up our orchestra, then we are reliant on the nervous system to act as our conductor, ensuring that the 'concerto of strength' is played at full volume and power. In fact, the nervous system and the musculoskeletal system are completely connected and embedded. Our brains send a signal down our spines, into a nerve, which takes it towards its target muscle. The endpoint is a neuromuscular junction that looks like tiny tentacles connected to the muscle fibre. This is literally the place in which our thoughts – 'I am going to stand up now' – become a reality, via an electrical signal that travels at incredible speed from our brains to the nerve endings controlling the thigh and glute muscles. The more neuromuscular junctions you have, the more effectively you can contract those muscles, which in turn means you can generate more force. In effect, the more muscle fibres you can contract, the stronger you will be.

As we will learn in Chapter 3, *how* we train will dictate the types of muscle fibres that our nerves will connect to and activate. But it's far more interesting than just the act of muscle contraction. We will also talk about how strength training can boost our nervous system, improving our balance and preventing us from falls. Research confirms that falls after the age of 65 are the leading causes of mortality due to injury and cost the NHS around £2 billion a year.[6,7,8] Broken bones or other injuries sustained in such falls often have the knock-on effect of immobility, leading to a spiralling loss of muscle mass and acceleration into frailty and vulnerability. Further, the nervous system plays a key role in our mood, rest, stress levels and how we perceive threat – which as we will learn in the coming chapters, may have profound consequences on our long-term ability to maintain our strength.

Connective tissue

Have you ever wondered why we tend not to recover as quickly or are stiffer for longer after exercise as we get older? Most of us have had the shock of experiencing stiff legs the morning after a long walk, bike ride, game of tennis or perhaps our children's sports day. I have lost count of the number of people I have seen in clinic a week after the parents' race with an injured body part (and ego).

Just as muscles age, so too do the more fibrous tendons and ligaments. Tendons and ligaments work together in an important partnership – our ligaments stabilise our joints and our tendons act as the bridge that connects our muscles to our bones. Both are essential elements in our ability to age well. Without these tissues in a strong state, we can expect injury, altered ability to move normally and higher chances of falling in older age.

So, it's important that we pay attention to these structures as we embark on our strength-building journey. But how many of us think of tendons in relation to strength training? Not many, I suspect. Instead, we are understandably likely to focus on the main characters – our muscles and bones – when we think about maintaining strength. However, maintaining elasticity and strength in our tendons is key. Unfortunately, these qualities lessen as we age. The fibres within them become more rigid, making them less able to transmit forces and in turn more prone to damage or injury.

When explaining the importance of our connective tissues to my clients, I use the example of a sailing yacht. Imagine the sails of a yacht with a rope in the corner of one sail. The sail represents the muscle and the rope is the tendon. If you do not have a rope that is able to handle the forces blowing on the sail a few things are going to happen. If your rope, or tendon, is weak, it will be stretched and strained by the force of the sail, giving rise to conditions like tendonitis (an inflammation of a tendon). Worse, you might suffer a tear that will put you out of action. Finally, if that rope is not securely attached to the boat, or in this case the bone, then all that force that is coming down it will be lost, and you risk pulling it completely from the bone. Happily, such rare events are preventable by paying attention to our long-term strength and flexibility.

One of the most recognisable signs of ageing in a person is how they move. They might be slower, look stiffer and be losing their ability to move normally. One of the factors affecting these ageing characteristics is again found in our connective tissues. Ligaments or tendons can physically shorten from disuse, which in turn leads to aches and pains, as well as reduced movement in our joints – ultimately decreasing the health of the cartilage in them.

If we allow our muscles to lose strength as we age, we will also lose it in our tendons. A classic outcome would be a joint or tendon injury if we were to participate in unaccustomed exercise, such as running for a train or in a parents' race on sports day. Therefore, it is sensible for those who haven't done much strength training in the past to spend longer initially building up their strength to allow more time for the tendons to adapt to the loading that this type of exercise entails. This is because a tendon takes longer to strengthen than a muscle. To this end, I have included a programme that will improve their function in Part 2 of this book. (See *Minimal Loading Programme* in Chapter 6.)

Bones

Our bones tell the story of our health. Have you ever watched a TV drama in which an osteologist (bone specialist) or archaeologist describes the type of life a person had, their level of health, injuries suffered, sorts of food they ate or how strong they were simply by examining their bones? In this case, fiction isn't far from the truth.

Depending on our long-term movements and habits, our bones will lay down certain lines in response to forces we are exposed to. The more dynamic or varied our movement, the more varied these lines will be, and consequently the better our bones' ability to deal with the stresses or strains we encounter throughout our lives. Those of us who do not move enough, or in the right way, risk weakening our bones' architectural integrity.

Variation in movement and force are medicine for our bones.

As an osteopathy student, I had to spend many hours in anatomy classes examining bones and was always mindful that I too was the owner of these marvels buried beneath my flesh. I was fascinated by the thought that I was laying down my own lines and patterns in response to the forces created through my daily activities. A skilled osteologist could look at the femur (thigh) bone, and with reasonable accuracy pinpoint what that person experienced in their lives, whilst also making assumptions about their work or exercise behaviours. They do this by looking out for tell-tale signs; for example, it is possible to determine that someone was sedentary due to minimal or mainly straight lines in the top of their femur. Often it is this region of bone that is prone to fracture in a fall. Conversely, the femur of an individual who was active and participated in weightbearing or dynamic activity would exhibit beautiful three-dimensional spiral lines, a clear indicator of their vitality and health. Bones that have moved more in life become stronger and are more able to absorb the forces generated in a fall without breaking. Being active in the right way produces incredible spiral structures that would not look out of place in an art gallery or an architect's drawing.

As we have learned, trips and falls in older age are the leading cause of death from accidents. Even if we have good balance and strength, all accidents can't be avoided, but if our bones are strong, most of the time we will be fine. As we age the strength of our bones declines in keeping with the amount of muscle we have. In fact, there is a relationship between the age-related loss of muscle mass and osteoporosis, a condition characterised by fragile or even brittle bones. Osteoporosis can also be driven by underlying medical conditions or poor diet, and in women is exacerbated by the effects of the menopause and declining oestrogen levels. Factors like not eating the right foods, drinking too much alcohol or smoking also increase our risk of developing this condition.

The factors not talked about as much include the lack of the right type of exercise and the subsequent effects on our skeleton. If we do not participate in regular strength training, combining it with a dynamic exercise such as running, we are not strengthening our bones as well as we could or think we are. It is only when we combine such activities that helpful forces are able to build the structural integrity of our bones. I can hear many runners shouting: 'This proves that running is sufficient to protect against osteoporosis!' and there is a degree of logic to this. But as I have explained previously, running is only doing half the job. Osteoporosis is closely associated with loss of muscle mass, so running alone will not protect us from it, as it tends to preserve mainly slow-twitch fibres. We need to combine running or other dynamic activities with strength training to gain maximal protection for our bones in older age, by building those fast-twitch fibres.

Exposing our bones to forces during strength training also acts as a wonderful stimulation for a stronger skeleton. The controlled compressive forces that strength training delivers stimulate specialist bone cells into manufacturing stronger bone, whilst also maintaining our fast-twitch fibres, both associated with protection against osteoporosis.

It is universally agreed that having a varied diet and taking part in a variety of different activities is positive for digestive system and brain health respectively. Experiencing a variety of *forces* is equally as beneficial for our bones. There are many applications of the phrase: 'our actions define us'; and this could not be truer for our bones.

Immune to ageing?

I am sure that not many people think about their ability to fight infections whilst strength-training, but it's a fact that preserving our muscle and strength also preserves our immune system.[9]

Maintaining our skeletal muscle bolsters our ability to respond to infection, so much so that I strongly support the concept of skeletal muscle as an 'immune organ'. Having a robust muscle mass provides a reservoir of amino acids, which helps our immune system to respond more quickly to germs and diseases. However, the presence of fat cells can compromise this immune response.

Fat cells cause inflammation which, when combined with the inflammation caused by viruses like Covid, often overwhelms our ability to fight an infection or indeed breathe efficiently. Fat cells infiltrate structures that are associated with our immune system, such as the spleen, muscle and bone marrow, diminishing the body's ability to respond to an infection. This combination is referred to as 'sarcopenic obesity', which represents the perfect storm for the long-term health of our muscles.[10] It is now clear that healthy skeletal muscle, free from the effects of fat cell infiltration, acts as an integral part of our immune response to both inflammation and infection.

By preserving our strength and maintaining a healthy weight in middle age and beyond, we can enhance our resilience against viruses and bacteria. This is particularly significant given the challenges experienced by the older generation during the pandemic and, indeed, every winter flu season.

2

Why Strength Matters

'Strength; The quality or state of being physically strong.'
The Oxford English Dictionary

f I were to ask you what your definition of strength was, what would you say? If we look at a typical dictionary listing, we find synonyms such as *stable, firm, tough, vigorous, robust* or my personal favourite: *welly*! Meanwhile, the antonyms are *weak, frail, brittle, breakable* and *vulnerable*. Which of these do you want to define you in older age? I ask because the amount of physical strength we have can define our quality of life. As we age, this influence becomes greater, until it is the dominant factor affecting our health and independence. Strength acts as a catch-all value that underpins many aspects of our lives, but its pivotal importance in our long-term physical health is underestimated by most.

Are you middle-aged and already exercising? What if I told you that you were probably not approaching it with the correct intensity or frequency to preserve that strength most effectively? Would you be surprised if I told you that by doing less overall or giving yourself permission to have rest days, you would in fact stay stronger for longer? No doubt this feels counter-intuitive to the 'work hard, play hard' narrative that has dominated attitudes to exercise over the last 40 years, but it's time we flipped the script.

A change in mindset

Many people have the erroneous notion that the only way to optimise fitness and strength is to train very hard ALL the time. This is usually as a response to the misplaced beliefs that training harder, longer and more often will lead to better strength or athletic gains. This pervasive message has seeped into gym culture, sports teams, military practices and many other areas within western culture, leading to unhelpful and often damaging long-term perceptions around fitness training. Everyday examples such as 'pain is weakness leaving the body', 'run it off', 'go hard or go home' and even 'sleep when you are dead' are just a few that I was personally familiar with. The truth is that for most of us, such motivational phrases just don't apply – and are especially dangerous in extremely physical careers such as the military, rescue, or elite sports teams. The levels of fitness seen in such groups are not sustainable over a lifetime and have the potential to negatively impact one's later life through injury or burnout. This is why we don't see 65-year-old marines or firefighters on the front line, or 70-year-olds competing with 20-year-olds in athletics events.

Why then would we expect optimal fitness gains as a middle-aged person if we adopt the training strategies of much younger, often elite groups?

Worryingly, it is often in those who are already exercising that we find a lack of awareness about how to approach strength training, or more relevant to us, how to train to preserve strength as we age. As a 50-year-old former firefighter, competitive rower, conditioning expert, osteopath and lifelong fitness enthusiast, my focus now is on exercise which helps me preserve as much later-life strength as possible. To come to this realisation, my midlife ego first had to accept that if I trained in the same way as 25-year-old me did, two things would happen. Firstly, I would not be able to move for about five or six days, and secondly, I would be diminishing my chances of older-age strength.

But what do I mean by this? Well, it might help if I explain my own strength journey and my more than 30-year relationship with exercise. At the age of 50, I had been training for years with the mindset of a much younger person striving for an elite level of fitness – I completely bought into the *work hard-train hard* philosophy. Successfully attaining a high level of physical fitness had, in many ways, defined who I was. The problem was that I was no longer this person. I was middle-aged, medically retired from the services, physically changed by injury, and was finding that my health had not improved as I was expecting it to in spite of the large amount of exercise I was doing. I was then approached to work on public health projects that focused on helping older people to preserve their strength and independence. This was the best thing that could have happened to me because the deeper I researched and the more I worked with clients, the more I realised that we should ignore the unhelpful motivational soundbites and instead engage with the facts of ageing and exercise. It became crystal clear that the route to better health is not to train harder, but to train smarter.

Exercise trends have fallen into unhelpful extremes. Either we don't place enough focus on exercise and live sedentary lifestyles, or we over-train using the wrong techniques. Even when people do try to start building up their strength, they often feel excluded from a gym setting, no longer identifying with the culture or feeling comfortable about exercising in this environment.

To help you zone in on your goals, perhaps ask yourself some questions:

- *How much exercise or physical activity do you do a week?*
- *What are your goals in getting stronger?* Perhaps you have a bucket list of things you want to do in later life? Why not write some of them down in the margins of this book and put a cross next to them if they are going to require you to be strong and fit. Be honest with yourself and consider if you are strong enough right now to get the most out of these activities. If not, how are you going to be strong enough in 20 or 30 years? This simple exercise can be a useful reality check, inviting you to consider whether you are taking your physical ability in later life for granted.
- *Are you doing nothing or less than the minimal recommended amounts of exercise?* You might not be aware of the dangers of inactivity (yet) but in any case, you cannot identify with people who are exercising.
- *Are you exercising, but have not prioritised strength training as essential to your long-term health?* You may be motivated to engage in activities that focus more on aerobic and endurance fitness

such as running or cycling. You might do a small amount of resistance training but will generally avoid trying an exercise that feels alien.

- *Are you participating in resistance training but not following a programme focusing on later-life strength preservation?* You may have more familiarity with strength training but are at risk of injury, fatigue and burnout – I was most definitely in this group.

Why start now? Physical over fiscal investment

How many of us are currently paying into savings plans, pensions pots or other financial schemes that we hope will afford us a good retirement? Perhaps we're saving up for the big trip we've always dreamed of. If you wrote some bucket list items in the margin above, I wonder if experiences like following the Inca trail, trekking to Everest base camp or walking in the Grand Canyon were included? What about just having the ability to walk around a new city and explore a museum that you've always wanted to visit? How about playing golf or taking the road trip that you've always wanted to experience? It is ironic that the physical strength required for a happy and healthy retirement often plays second fiddle to financial stability. Yet without physical strength, no amount of money can help us improve our situation. Financial stability will not matter if we haven't protected our postural stability. Irrespective of the promises of some sections of the 'longevity industry', there is currently no magic wand to make you stronger. The truth is we must work for strength to preserve our muscle and apply that effort in the most efficient ways, at the most effective stages of our lives. To borrow a common phrase, it really is true that *health* is *wealth*.

Now take your bucket list and copy it into the shaded area opposite, remembering to add new ones and cross old ones off as you complete them.

Your strength bucket list

1. ....

2. ....

3. ....

4. ....

5. ....

Understanding strength, power and muscular endurance

When I talk about strength, I am referring to our ability to maximally contract a muscle or muscle group and the force that this generates. An everyday example of strength might be getting up from a chair. For some people, this simple movement might represent a maximal effort on their part. To achieve this, they must be able to successfully contract their leg and thigh muscles to generate the force needed to overcome their body weight and the effects of gravity. For others, this will be relatively easy to accomplish. You can get an accurate measure of a person's grip force by using a dynamometer – a handheld device with a handle to squeeze and a display that tells you how many pounds per square inch their squeeze applied.

Power is the speed at which we can maximally contract a muscle or group of muscles. In the standing-from-a-chair scenario, someone who is able to get up faster has generated more power. Returning to the grip dynamometer, several people might have exactly the same result, but it is the person who achieved their maximal grip reading the fastest who is the most powerful. In other words, their ability to generate their maximal strength was faster, which as will learn later, can literally save our lives when we are older.

We need strength and speed to generate power.

Muscular endurance is the ability to perform multiple submaximal contractions of a muscle or muscle group. In the case of our example, this might be how many times someone can perform a sit-to-stand test before they become tired.

Think back to our strength reservoir. If the level is too low, we will not have the raw material to improve our muscular endurance or power. Muscular endurance and power are fed and maintained by our strength, not the other way around. We need to follow different patterns when training in order to achieve improvement in the specific areas of strength, power and muscle.

How many of us have focused on going to the gym or playing sports when planning our exercise routine? This will have been doing us lots of good in terms of joint mobility, cardiovascular health, metabolic health, and muscular endurance. But have we been improving strength? To a certain extent we have, but not as efficiently as you might have thought. It is true that at easy or moderate levels of effort, regular resistance training can help to offset some of the age-related effects of muscle loss. So even if you are not willing or able to increase the intensity of the training, you will be doing some good. However, I believe we should prepare to have as much strength in our reservoir as possible, because this will increase our chances of recovering and returning to normal following an unforeseen illness, injury or life event. Just like a boxer preparing for a long fight, we must train with the mindset of being strong, not just in the early or middle rounds, but in the later rounds too. Especially if we want to win!

Does size matter?

If there was ever a time when we could legitimately ask out loud if size matters, now is that time! Those who are solely focused on increasing muscle size (hypertrophy) through training, such as bodybuilders, often achieve significant changes in strength as well as size. However, many bodybuilders, although stronger than an untrained individual, are more concerned with aesthetics than preserving strength. Increases in size are also seen with strength training, and to a lesser extent with power training and lesser still with muscular endurance activities. Any increase in muscle size stands us in good stead for long-term health but only if we have trained that muscle to be strong and powerful in all the directions we need it to be. In other words, there is nothing wrong with gaining strong, powerful muscle that is ready to function in our everyday lives.

It is an urban myth that bodybuilders are healthy. Although currently strong and owners of impressive muscle mass, they are not typically able to maintain this into older age. When was the last time you saw an 80-year-old bodybuilder? I guess you never have, as such an intense regime is not normally sustainable into older age. Aside from the long-term dangers of performance-enhancing substances, I believe that this type of exercise actually begins to have a negative effect on long-term health, similar to the over-training effects previously discussed.

As to the question of whether size matters, the fact that we lose strength at a faster rate than muscle mass suggests that it is not quite that simple. Since power deteriorates at an even faster rate than strength, we need to participate in activities that draw on the pivotal relationship between our nervous system and our muscles. More in Chapter 3 and Part 2 on how strength training can keep this relationship healthy. Needless to say, we need to keep both our muscles and the nervous system controlling them in good condition to maximise our strength and health in older age.

Getting stronger

The process involved in getting stronger is fascinating. Like most other living tissues, a muscle requires stimulus to change. It simply will not improve if it is not under stress or tension. If given no stimulation, as with a chronically inactive person, muscles will literally wither away. Within the structure of a skeletal muscle fibre, we find actin and myosin proteins that respond to the physical stress and tension that resistance training delivers. Stress in this context means working our muscle fibres against a force – like pushing, pulling, lifting, carrying and lowering either your own body weight or equipment such as weights, to act as the resistance. At home, this might look like press-ups, squats, pull-ups or dips, use of bands or other equipment. At a gym, this might also include machines.

The interesting thing here is that it is not just the muscles working against resistance, adapting and growing stronger. It is the interaction between the nerves and the muscle fibres that can make a difference. The more we use resistance training, the more we can elicit beneficial changes in both our nerves and muscles. The entire nervous system will adapt in some way in response to strength training. But more relevant to this section, the stimulation of resistance training recruits more motor endplates (the endpoint of the nerve that controls muscle contraction), laying the way for a chemical response that signals the muscle fibres to adapt. It's a bit like an irrigation system on a veg patch; regular watering stimulates larger vegetables. In the same way, regular resistance training stimulates growth of our skeletal muscle.

Depending on the type of training, the heads of the myosin molecules – the motor proteins found in our muscles – become larger in response to that stimulation. If you are training for endurance, they will only grow a little. If, however, you are training to build and maintain muscle mass, strength and power, the change will be more significant. It is this myosin head enlargement that drives the observable outward size increase of a muscle.

Our long-term goal should be to preserve our muscle mass, strength and power so that we have strong joints and a healthy posture deep into older age.

There's more about the perfect programme for balancing our long-term muscle, strength and power needs in the Foundation 10 Movements in Part 2.

One of the common concerns I hear, especially from women, is about the fear of looking too bulky. However, there's no need to worry. It is true that some subtle increases in muscle size might accompany strength training, but by middle age, our days of significant size gain are behind us. We are talking about gaining some muscle, getting as strong as we can and then working to preserve that strength into older age. It is possible to become stronger without any overt changes in muscle size. In later-life health, overall strength is far more important than having huge muscles.

But if (like most of us) you happen to be motivated by aesthetics as well as longevity, then I guarantee that strength training is the best way to improve our overall shape and tone those areas of our bodies that are more prone to the effects of gravity!

Your personal relationship with strength

The level of strength that can be attained will vary according to the individual. Your own strength potential is as unique as your life experiences. Even someone who has built up a good level of strength in their forties and maintained it into middle age, will of course see it declining over time, as their hormonal levels start to decrease. However, if they continue regular strength training into older age, they will be rewarded by staying well above the threshold of inactivity-related disability and frailty.

How we do this will be dictated by our mindset. We must hold the belief that we too can be strong and independent as an older person. The strong, athletic, older people I have had the privilege of working with hold this mindset. They all believed that they would be strong and healthy in older age, with many of them using positive affirmations to motivate themselves. The language we use to describe ourselves to others and indeed speak to ourselves has the potential to shape our beliefs and behaviours. Common phrases such as 'taking it easy', 'winding down' or 'relaxing' in retirement, or 'being put out to pasture' when older no doubt originate from a desire to be kind, or to look after someone. But these terms can have a knock-on effect on the way we actually behave – presenting inactivity as a benefit of finally retiring.

Think for a minute about some of the phrases that have become embedded in our cultural vocabulary. There are many examples that

seriously deter people from keeping strong and healthy in older age –
'over the hill', 'past one's prime', 'long in the tooth' – they all present
ageing as a descent into a less-positive stage of life. Even the more
encouraging language we use to celebrate those people who keep active
in older age – 'fit as someone half their age', 'you would not believe how
old they are!' – all paint the picture that keeping fit is a rarity.

It is important to remember that these people do not possess any
kind of advantage; they are not genetically predisposed to remain
strong and powerful; rather somewhere along the line they have made
the decision, perhaps in middle age, to continue doing what they
enjoyed doing. We can all be older athletic versions of ourselves; we
simply need to believe it is achievable and continue to exercise.

My hope is that by engaging with this knowledge you will begin
your journey to a stronger old age by starting to do the same. Even if
the rest of the world does not share our positive outlook, let's prove that
narrative wrong.

3

Why the Nervous System Matters

'Our bodies are our gardens – our wills are our gardeners.'
William Shakespeare

I n 1932, Sir Charles Sherrington won the Nobel prize for a lifetime's work on the human nervous system. He famously called the motor neurones of the spinal cord 'the final common pathway', meaning that movement of a muscle is dependent on a signal from a nerve. Put simply, our muscles only work if our nerves do. Given that a sizable percentage of our health in older age is dependent on healthy skeletal muscle, it is vital to learn what controls, excites, calms, heals and activates this tissue. Introducing: our nervous system.

How we learn to move and control our bodies has always been a source of fascination for me. As a clinician, I have assessed how thousands of patients move. Sometimes I have been able to make this assessment before even meeting a patient in person. From our clinician's room, I often see a patient walking to reception. From this distance, I can usually form an accurate picture of their history of injury or what exercise they have done. Even before they enter the door of my clinic, I can visualise which muscle groups they will need to strengthen and how I can help them improve. Most of us go through our days taking the most everyday activities for granted, such as walking, running, or indeed typing. How about the act of reading, in which the tracking of your eyes across the page is similar to that of someone watching a tennis match? All these movements, however small, are the end output of a nerve signal that originated in your brain, journeying down your spine and into a nerve, and on to its target muscle. The end of the nerve, called a motor end plate, acts as a spark plug in activating that muscle to move.

For some years now, therapists have observed the benefits to patients of being actively engaged in their own recovery. By better understanding the nervous system and its part in building strength, I hope that you will be primed to embrace your own process of becoming older and stronger.

The vine of movement

If you have been lucky enough to visit vineyards in countries such as France or Italy, you have likely enjoyed the atmosphere and hopefully sampled a little wine. When I see a vine, my osteopath brain sees a natural system that feeds, nurtures, signals and stimulates growth – just like our nervous system.

If a vine is established and thick, it is better able to produce good grapes. Just as it is impossible to have healthy grapes without a healthy vine, so too is it impossible to have healthy muscles without a healthy nervous system. The mind and body are irrevocably linked.

When first researching the nervous system during my injury recovery, I was struck by how powerful having a better understanding of it can be, and how it can inform how we live, train, rest and recover. Looking at some of the ways it manifests in our movement can also help us to diagnose certain conditions and make sense of the process of ageing. I'm sure you will have noticed that older people often move slowly, even when performing simple tasks like getting their wallet out to pay for their shopping. While this slowing can be a symptom of underlying neurological disease, more frequently it is due to a decrease in certain types of muscle fibres, leading to a decline in fine control when performing everyday tasks, like paying for shopping. Remember when I asked you to stand on one leg for 10 seconds? This is another real-time demonstration of the relationship between the nervous system and our muscles, with the length of time we can do this indicating how healthy that relationship is.

When explaining this concept to older clients or patients, I often say that the end of the nerve is, in a practical sense, like a door from one system to another. In this case, from the nervous to the musculoskeletal system. This door, from the mysterious world of our thoughts, transforms our intentions into movement and action. This is the mind connecting to the body.

Testing the connection

There is a handy exercise I use to test what someone's journey to getting strong will look like. It relies on the implicit relationship between our ability to control a muscle and the potential to get that muscle stronger. First, find a safe space, and then close your eyes. Whilst standing, sitting or lying down, focus your mind on the muscles on the front of your thighs, known as the quadriceps, or quads for short. Try to contract only those muscles as hard as you can without moving any other part of your leg. Can you contract those muscles to the point where they feel they might cramp? This point is maximal contraction. Can you contract only your target muscle group without affecting any others? Chances are you did quite well with the quads, because we generally use them most of the time and therefore have good control of them.

Now try to do the same with the muscles of the back of your thighs or hamstrings. How did this one go? If contracting one muscle group is harder than the other, it means that it will take more time to get stronger. It takes practice to embed movement patterns in our brains and spinal cords whilst improving local nerve function to the muscle group in question. Now return to the exercise and slowly try to isolate and contract the muscles of the chest or perhaps the small muscles of your shoulder blades.

Everyone will have areas that are easier to contract and others that are more difficult. In my clinic, I use this exercise as a starting point in someone's strength journey because it nicely highlights the mind–body connection. Movement in the body is achieved through the brain, spinal cord and peripheral nervous system working together to activate our muscles. The same system also drives the development of strength. We all have different muscle distributions, depending on our histories of exercise, injury, age, sex, nutrition and genetics – all of which can influence our strength. Helpfully, in most cases, increased use of a given muscle group will be a win-win, serving the dual purpose of improving both our neurological and muscular systems.

Proprioception (body sense)

Practice of any new skill is mediated in our nervous system and relies on the feedback that sensors in our muscles and joints relay back to our brains. This type of feedback is commonly referred to as 'proprioception', which is a term that was first coined by our friend Sir Charles Sherrington in 1893. This is how we know what positions our bodies are in at any given time. We are continually receiving real-time feedback from our muscles and joints via specialist nerve receptors, called mechanoreceptors, which supply information to us when we move. As we age, if we are not mobile or active, this feedback can decrease.

To test your proprioception skills, I'd like you to close your eyes and try to sense your thigh muscles. What position is your knee in? How tense are your muscles? How well you can differentiate this information demonstrates how efficiently your innate sense of your body is working. This is important because the better such connections, the better you will be at learning new movements and the more likely you will be to move efficiently. But don't worry if this is not easy to begin with. You can improve this skill with practice. Our nervous system is a superhighway of communication that dictates how we move and keeps us safe.

Muscle fibres in ageing – strength and power

As mentioned in Chapter 1, we have three main types of skeletal muscle fibres which are accompanied by specialised nerve motor endplates: 'slow twitch', 'fast twitch' and 'difficult-to-reach'. Everyday tasks that are relatively easy to perform are more dependent on slow-twitch fibres, for moderate to hard activity that requires increased speed or strength, we use our fast-twitch and difficult-to-reach types.

Most muscles have a mix of all fibre types, but this can vary depending on which area of the body we are looking at, our genetic predisposition and our history of exercise. This means that a muscle is usually distributed with a fibre type most suited to the job in hand. For instance, muscles that are working all the time, such as those that support our posture, need to be able to work for prolonged periods without getting tired. The Soleus muscle in the lower leg is a good example. Situated behind the knee, it works with other muscles in this region when we're running, walking or standing. It is the primary leg muscle used to maintain standing posture and it prevents us from swaying forward when upright. Because of this, it has a higher percentage of slow-twitch fibres than any other muscle.

As outlined in Chapter 1, our slow-twitch fibres are what we use for everyday activities or endurance exercise. They are well supplied with blood vessels and are very difficult to exhaust. People who only participate in such endurance exercise will have a much higher proportion of slow-twitch than fast-twitch fibres. When working with endurance-focused individuals, the first thing I ask them to do is start strength training in order to engage with and maintain their fast-twitch muscle. Conversely, I get patients who have focused on weight training to incorporate cardiovascular (endurance) training into their exercise plans to ensure good heart and lung function, whilst also building mitochondria in the muscle. (Mitochondria are tiny powerhouses inside cells that are involved in releasing energy from food.)

Depending on the type of exercise, a signal will be triggered locally that leads to adaptation within the muscle fibres. The activity we are doing will dictate which muscle fibres are activated and the degree of adaptation they achieve. Unfortunately, going for a gentle jog is not enough to improve the function of the fibres involved with our strength or power. That would be like dialling the operator and asking for a long-distance call, only to be put through to the wrong country.

Using running as an example: if we go for a jog, we will be using slow-twitch fibres. If we then find a hill and run up it repeatedly at pace, we will be using our fast-twitch fibres. If we push ourselves even harder by sprinting up the hill or carrying something heavy on our backs, we will be using our difficult-to-reach fibres. We need to be specific in both our exercise selection and the intensity we work at, to make sure we are developing and maintaining strength and power most effectively. If instead we are doing a strength-training exercise, such as a squat, we activate slow-twitch fibres. As squatting becomes more difficult, say after maintaining the position for 30 seconds, we begin to recruit our fast-twitch fibres. The longer we continue with the exercise, the harder it will become to perform, leading to the activation of the difficult-to-reach fibres. In very general terms, this is true for any strength training exercise. As the difficulty of the exercise is increased, either via additional resistance (from the amount of weight) or from increasing the time your muscle is under tension, the types of fibres used will change from simple to more complex, i.e. from slow to fast and finally difficult-to-reach.

We tend to have lots of slow- and fast-twitch fibres because, as humans, we spend most of our time in either easy or moderately easy physical situations. In fact, there is some preliminary research that seems to support what many coaches and individuals have observed during training for many years. Specifically, that some fibres perform a kind of *hybrid* role, hedging towards more endurance or strength characteristics depending on what exercise we are doing.[1] So, if you think you are more suited to only one type of training, think again! Our bodies will adapt to what we ask them to do.

In daily life, it is our fast-twitch fibres that are activated first, for example when we stumble, because we need to rapidly reach out to save ourselves or quickly correct our foot position. Difficult-to-reach fibres earn their name because we use them only once we have used the other fibres in our bank. The challenge with difficult-to-reach fibres is – you guessed it – to reach them. As we know from Chapter 1, in the later stages of life, both types of fast-twitch fibres are lost at a faster rate than the slow-twitch type.[2] The outcome of decreasing levels of fast-twitch fibres is a slowing of walking speed, a reduction in the size and strength of the fibres that remain, and a decline in fine motor control that is so often associated with lack of confidence. These issues are difficult to reverse after long periods of inactivity, even if you have once been strong. The key message here is that once we have made an effort to start strength training, there are huge later-life advantages to continuing it. Even if we are adapting how we strength-train as we age, continuing to use these fibres will keep them, and the nerves that activate them, very much alive.

Intentional power!

Strong, powerful muscles are a key ingredient of living our best lives in older age. This is because faster powerful movement is generated by our fast-twitch fibres, the loss of which predisposes us to frailty, falls, fracture and ill health. Luckily, it is completely possible to maintain these fibres with the correct type of training.

Simply put, power = strength x speed: meaning the faster we can contract a muscle, the greater the power produced. The challenge is that most of us will stop exercising, including strength training, as soon as we feel our muscles aching slightly, thus failing to utilise our difficult-to-reach fibres. In doing so, we risk falling into a trap where we incorrectly think we have a well-rounded strength programme. That is not to say we need to embrace the pain in every workout by always pushing to our extremes – far from it. But if we occasionally push ourselves by adopting exercise that includes short, sharp bursts of challenging work, we will ensure that we activate all our fibre types. This can include any element of your normal strength-training routine, for example a press-up or a squat, but with the added difficulty of trying to do it more rapidly.

If you are thinking that remaining powerful into older age is unrealistic, just seek out the veteran groups at running clubs or seniors who are still playing football, tennis, basketball or touch rugby. I guarantee that among their number there will be some men and women who would give the average middle-aged person a run for their money.

I expect very few of you will have seen people training for sprints in their seventies or eighties. However, those sprinters who have consistently trained from their youth into older age have distinct advantages over people of a similar age who are inactive. Amazingly, these older sprinters have maintained both types of their fast-twitch fibres and have protected both the size and power capacity of their muscles.[3] They can also expect to have a greater ability to generate power compared to a sedentary group, with some being able to perform a standing jump to twice (yes, twice!) the height achieved by someone of the same age who is sedentary. We already know that we need to have enough strength to generate power, and that power is a measure of how quickly you can generate force in a muscle or muscle group.

But what really matters is your intention during repeated attempts to move more quickly against resistance. Even if you do not manage to push, pull, lift or jump with greater speed, if your intention is to increase speed by repetition of an exercise or movement, then there will still be the potential to improve power.[4] Improvements in our nervous system, from repeated attempts to be more powerful, lead to an increase in the speed, quality and subsequent control of muscle contraction. As with learning other skills, the most important factor for becoming more powerful is the *practice* of trying to be more powerful. As to the exact mechanism of how our intention alone can lead to more power, this remains somewhat mysterious. However, the power of our thoughts, visualisation, intention and indeed expectations can all be useful tools in our strength journey.

Prevention over treatment

If you have ever done any kind of rehabilitation exercise that involved balancing on one leg, you were probably doing it with the end goal of improving an injured ligament or joint. But you were also engaging your entire nervous system, not merely the ligament in question. Life teaches us that we are highly likely to perform this type of exercise if we know it will improve a specific region or body part following an injury. In our culture, doing exercise to *recover* appears to be more acceptable than doing it to *prevent* injury. Rehabilitation versus pre-habilitation.

Speaking as a former firefighter, much of our focus was on prevention. Prevention of a fire was always better than fighting it, 100% of the time. However, it is well known that implementing prevention strategies in any setting is a difficult sell, because people tend not to engage with an ongoing issue until it becomes a real and immediate problem in their lives. How many times do people install a fire or burglar alarm after a house fire or after being burgled? Fear or upset can be great motivators for change. However, in the case of older-age strength, we need to understand that you can't start working on building power and strength in your older age and expect to undo years of detraining. If you have fallen or tripped and then decided to turn over a new leaf, as is often the case, your improvement will be limited by your age when you start. Far better to turn that leaf now *before* it becomes a real problem in later life.

Strength as a skill to master

The process of becoming physically stronger is much like learning a new skill or sport. When we strength-train, we engage many of the same mechanisms that we would when we learn to ride a bike, swim or even play the piano. It is a universal rule that skills that require movement will take many hours to master. When we see Lang Lang play, his fingers appear to flow effortlessly over the piano keys and we are awestruck. Perhaps, like me, you watched Jonny Wilkinson's winning drop kick in the 2003 Rugby World Cup final and were amazed by his ability to perform such a precise movement under incredible pressure. The truth is that both Lang Lang and Jonny Wilkinson had been obsessively practising for thousands of hours. For both, this repeated practice led to adaptation within the nervous system. If we revisit the vine/nervous system idea, regular resistance-training practice grows the thickness of our vines, maintaining and optimising the pathway for our nerve signals to travel through whilst maintaining our muscle strength. The thicker the vine, the stronger we will be in older age. But it is not enough just to initially improve our strength via resistance training. We must continue to include regular strength work in our exercise regime. Not doing so would be like spending years growing a vineyard then letting it wither away before you get to enjoy the vintage.

A stronger sense of self and strengthening the brain

Our sense of our own bodies, the awareness of the component parts of our physical selves, is in the frontal part of the brain – the somatosensory cortex. How we move in life shapes the way this part of the brain develops. The more we use certain muscles, the better the level of detail contained in the brain about those muscles. This is useful in our quest to retain later-life strength because greater brain detail means improved control of movement and increased exercise efficiency. If you are Lang Lang, you will have more intricate detail in the sensory cortex region involved with the hands, fingers and thumbs. In the case of Jonny Wilkinson, the region of cortex for his kicking foot would be more detailed than for his non-kicking foot. This representation of the body within the brain, known as the sensory homunculus, will adapt and respond to regular movements in our lives. If you spend more time sitting down, your sense of self will be as someone who sits, and you will be training your brain and in turn your body to be simply rather good at sitting. However, if you engage in exercise and in regular strength-based training, you are teaching your brain and body to be really good at moving, in turn creating your sense of self as someone who is strong. Part 2 will show you how to turn yourself into the strong version of you.

One initial insight into the long-term benefits of strength training came from the unlikely source of computer science. Researchers at the Alan Turing Institute analysed data from subjects using strength equipment. Their conclusions supported the evidence of many people working in rehabilitation and strength conditioning, namely that the benefits of engaging in exercise over longer periods of time will last for longer than those gained over a short term.[5] This concept is similar to the theory of 'muscle memory' and the dangers of relying on former glories, or in this case, former strength levels that we touched on in the introduction. Experts are still unsure if prior training can help us if we return to building muscle after a prolonged period of inactivity. There are broadly two main camps focused on the actions of our bodies during strength training: the muscle camp and the nervous system camp. The muscle camp argue that in building a muscle fibre once, we have a long-term advantage, even if it decreases in size over time due to lack of use. This is possibly due to the presence of the muscle nuclei, which power the building of new muscle fibre. They are created through strength training and seem to be preserved, even when the muscle fibre decreases in size. If we return to our sailing yacht analogy, it's a bit like building your racing sail, but also investing in an on-board racing computer – *nucleus* - that ensures you achieve an optimal performance from your sails. If you are inactive and you revert back to a normal non-racing sail, you will still have your racing computer ready and waiting until you start to strengthen your racing sails again. Needless to say, we shouldn't become complacent, because if we were once strong but fall into inactivity for too long, there is a risk that the fibres and the nerve endings will never be the same again and you'll be stuck with a great racing computer operating a set of dinghy sails.

The nervous system camp has another theory. It is generally accepted that there is adaptation going on in the nervous system as we get stronger, which is preserved even when we are inactive for prolonged periods afterwards. Those who were once strong can regain some strength rapidly, following inactivity, even in the absence of increasing muscle size. This indicates that the re-acquisition of strength is in part driven by retained nervous system adaptations to strength training.[6] It is also a real-life example of how the collaboration between nerves and muscles can determine our strength. So when it comes to the role of our nervous system in strength, the term 'muscle memory' couldn't be more relevant. The brain and spinal cord movement patterns created by strength training are long-lasting. That said, as we know from earlier in this chapter, we really don't want to be inactive for too long and risk our fast-twitch fibres being downgraded to slow!

It is also clear that we can draw on the memory of the process of improving some aspect of physical performance, such as becoming stronger. Positive memory is an especially powerful tool when revisiting an activity if we have previously overcome what seemed like daunting physical challenges. Having confidence in your own ability boosts your trust in the process of physical improvement.

Don't skip leg day

How people want to look can determine what body areas they choose to strengthen. Personally, I'm not a big fan of the skinny-jeans look for men for two reasons. One is, aesthetically, it's not always the most flattering look for a middle-aged man, but also and more importantly, it isn't particularly healthy, as skinny legs can be a signifier of a lack of strength in that area. Research found that in older people, the signal travelling down the spinal cord from the brain decreases when it comes to the nerves of the thighs or legs, meaning it is harder to maintain the strength of our lower limbs than upper limbs.[7] This is relevant to later-life strength and independence because as we've explored, lower-limb function is often a decisive factor in assessing an older individual's ability to live independently. The phrase 'skipping leg day' is used in gym culture to describe a person who chooses not to strengthen the muscles in their lower extremities for a variety of reasons. Although it might be funny to think that an entire generation has grown up trying to have a strong upper body with subsequently weaker legs, in reality this isn't a good idea.

NASA, the NFL and lessons from sport

It is not uncommon for scientific studies that were originally meant to help a specific group of people to end up benefiting a much larger population. A great example of this is the NASA research that took place in the 1990s in which scientists examined the dyslexia-type effect that zero gravity was having on space shuttle crews. They designed a programme of sensory exercises to alleviate these symptoms, which not only helped astronauts on future missions but proved highly effective in helping dyslexic adults and children around the world.

A more fitting example regarding the importance of strength and movement, and this time on land, can be seen in the lessons taken from the American National Football League (NFL). The NFL has some of the most powerful, fast and talented athletes on the planet. Speed, power, precise movement and physical strength are currency in their world, and yet, perhaps counter-intuitively, some giants of this sport have spent many hours trying to go slower rather than faster in training. Legendary American football coach Tom Martinez recognised the importance of the nervous system in relation to physical performance: 'It's not how fast you can do it. It's how slowly you can do it correctly.'[8] What he was talking about was the ability of our nervous system to control movement. Increased strength and power in the skeletal muscles are meaningless without the control to safely apply that force to a given task and indeed stop again safely. Imagine running fast and not being able to stop, kicking a ball and not being able to adjust your strike if the ball moves at the last minute or, for our purposes, an older person not being able to save themselves from a fall. The reason this is so important is that in life we can't always rely on momentum to complete a movement – we also need control.

In my own clinical practice, one of the first things I do in an assessment is ask a patient to stand in front of a large mirror and perform a slow full squat. Assessing the muscles over their full range of motion and the subtle adjustments being made at the person's spine, hip, and knee joints provides a rich seam of information about that individual's true strength, joint range, proprioception, foot–ankle stability, balance and mind–body connection. If I had asked them to do the same assessment as fast as possible, it would have been meaningless, because gravity and momentum mask any issues in coordination, muscle strength and balance. The very same principle that defined Tom Martinez's approach to working with NFL players can inform ours to older-age strength. If you feel, as is very common, that one side is weaker than another in any movement – or that a specific joint lacks stability – try moving slowly and observe any obvious differences. In doing so, you will get a realistic picture of your joint range, muscle control and proprioception, which will consequently serve as a useful tool in deciding what movements or muscle groups you need to focus on.

Watching and visualising exercise can make you stronger

Sticking to the world of sport, when we see Olympic weightlifters banging their chests or leg muscles before lifting, I wonder if they realise that they are engaging with a neurological mechanism that can help them lift. As well as psyching themselves up, the weightlifters are making sure their brains know which muscle is about to be used and reinforcing the message with touch. But before we start banging our chests before our workouts, you'll be pleased to hear we can achieve the same effect another way. As discussed, simply thinking about a body part can help improve our mind's ability to control it. Contracting the muscle before you exercise it will also work well, as will applying elastic kinesio tape to a particular area. It works by letting our brains know that we are about to use a particular muscle or joint. In turn, our nervous system has time to prepare to move, brace or protect a joint from injury. We are essentially giving a 'heads-up' to our nervous system to get ready for action or to be careful. I have successfully used this 'soft-taping' method many times with athletes following injury because it increases their awareness of the taped area. The point here is that we can use these techniques to improve the mind–body connection and in turn our ability to keep safe and strong.

Our mind–body connection is so powerful that we can often activate parts of the brain associated with certain movements simply by watching others move or thinking about those movements ourselves.[9] There are sets of motor and sensory cells within the brain that are used whenever we move, for example from sitting to standing. The amazing thing about these cells, known as mirror neurons, is that around 20% of them are still activated if we merely watch someone else standing up. Simply observing or visualising movement can build our own ability to perform certain motions.

Often, we will say that a sports person is 'in the zone' before they compete. This is because they are visualising competing to their highest standard and most importantly, winning. We now know that they are warming up their nervous system, just as they also warm up their muscles. Deep visualisation can also reap real benefit within the nervous system by developing neural pathways without physically engaging in the activity. But this is not an excuse not to do the exercise! What I am saying here is that if you are new to strength, why not use the power of the mind and nervous system to help motivate you? Visualise a strength session the day before, when you wake up that day, or just before your session. Return to the concept of the internal vine and visualise it lighting up and charging your muscles with the impulse to move, so that when you come to take part in the exercise, it may well feel far easier than expected.

Our beliefs and expectations dictate our strength

Often the biggest obstacles stopping us from starting and then sticking to an exercise programme are our own thoughts and how we see ourselves. Belief in our ability to exercise can have a dramatic impact on performance. In his book, *The Expectation Effect*, David Robinson explores the power that lies within our expectations. If we have positive expectations about our older age and physical abilities, then we are more likely to achieve positive health in older age.[10] This phenomenon is borne out by the attitudes shared by older generations living in Blue Zones, as well as older sprinters and sports enthusiasts. Strength should be no different – anyone who is serious about being a stronger version of themselves needs to start by believing that this is possible and achievable. Once you believe it, you should start to use visualisation to imagine an older version of yourself who is strong; continuing to strength-train and living their best life. For sports people, it is natural to use positive thought or visualisation to gain an advantage in their field. For those of us whose goal is to retain as much strength as possible in later life, there is no reason not to adopt the same approach. It has been shown that such strategies, far from being passive, are neurologically active processes that can help improve our performance in exercise and everyday life.

Relaxation, rest and breathing can make you stronger

Strength training and building the relationship between our nervous system and muscles are clearly vital in fighting frailty in older age. But it's equally as important to look at what happens once the exercise has stopped. Becoming stronger is also about resting, relaxing and breathing, to allow ourselves time to recharge.

You may have heard about the fight or flight response to stress, also known as our sympathetic system. This system responds to stressful or dangerous situations by diverting blood flow to our brain and muscles, allowing us to use these muscles optimally in these situations.

However, there is another system that gets much less attention but is no less important – the parasympathetic system. It functions in the opposite way to the sympathetic system, and is used when we repair tissues, replenish nutrients and excrete waste. For strength training, the quicker we can get into this state of replenishment and repair after exercise, the better for our general health and long-term strength. (More on how these systems can affect our strength in Chapter 4.)

If you were asked to make a list containing what you felt was essential in maximising your chances of enjoying older-age strength, how likely would you be to include rest, relaxation, sleep and mindfulness?

If we are not resting, sleeping or eating well, we stand little chance of preserving later-life strength. Our nervous system needs to switch easily between sympathetic and parasympathetic modes to optimise the entire process of exercise. Recognising the value of your down time and giving yourself permission to rest your body for recharging is imperative for improving strength. We need to become better at relaxing post-exercise, for example stretching whilst concentrating on controlled breathing. Many elite athletes, military forces and emergency services follow such post-workout protocols, allowing their body to return to a restorative state as rapidly as possible.

Try box breathing
Breath in for the count of four
Hold your breath for the count of four
Exhale for the count of four
Hold your breath for the count of four.
Repeat 3-4 times.

Whilst you do this, try focusing on the outward movement of your lower ribs as you inhale to encourage more diaphragmatic breathing.

Such breathing patterns have been shown to help in switching from a sympathetic to a parasympathetic state. The diaphragm is itself skeletal muscle, primarily involved with respiration, but it is also central to many exercises in which we need to control our breathing. For example, to 'brace' our bodies, when lifting in everyday life or strength-training. Breath work also plays a central role in breathing efficiency and relaxation because of its link to the parasympathetic nervous system.

Putting our minds to strength

Like skeletal muscle, our nervous system responds to new experiences, challenges and controlled stress. In the extremes of performance, it might be that you develop incredible athleticism and balance as a martial artist or gymnast. In the arts, you might develop awe-inspiringly precise control of hand movement when painting or playing an instrument. At the other end of performance within normal daily life, if we do not pay attention to the nervous system, we become vulnerable to balance issues, begin to move differently, sacrifice precious fast-twitch fibres, and lose confidence in anything movement-related. To borrow a common phrase, if we 'put our minds to it', not only will it help us activate our skeletal muscles, but also give us enhanced balance that will decrease our chances of falling and help us move more efficiently. Improvements in our frontal cortex and spinal cord will effectively lead to energy savings because our movements will be smoother and more efficient. Regular exercise that activates all three types of our muscle fibres will reinforce our neuromuscular connections, preserving later-life strength and our ability to generate power. Finally, and just as importantly, remember that maintaining a positive outlook on later-life strength is more likely to make each of us a stronger older person.

During an era in which many aspects of neurology remained beyond our understanding, the Nobel Science Committee recognised Sir Charles Sherrington's work.[11] Modern science has now validated and built upon Sherrington's observations about the nervous system, leading to insights that can help us achieve the ultimate goal of this book: creating a strong, powerful and athletic older you.

4

Evolutionary Strength

'Experience is the teacher of all things.'
Julius Caesar

I f you share my love of history documentaries, you may already appreciate how we can deepen our understanding of ourselves by discovering how differently we lived in the past, particularly looking back to a time when our very distant ancestors walked the planet. I am not talking about searching for clues in 20,000-year-old fossilised bones, but rather if we want to understand modern humans, looking at our biological systems and behaviours in the context of our more ancient or primitive selves. Because whether we like it or not, 'primitive' us is often in charge of our day-to-day life, and the clash between modern and primitive living has the potential to negatively impact our long-term strength if left unchecked.

The human species is an upright, movement-based organism that has evolved and survived not by being sedentary and weak but by actively engaging with its environment – all of which requires physical robustness and strength. Physical inactivity directly contravenes ancient innate movement and survival instincts that have been inherited by our modern-day biology. As such, the complexity and beauty in our ability to heal, sense, adapt, respond and learn are evidence of our evolutionary journey.

If you can't see how evolution influences our everyday lives, have you ever walked into a room and forgotten what you went in there for? The common phenomenon known as the 'doorway effect' is said by some researchers to indicate the need of our ancient ancestors to focus their attention when passing through a threshold, to guard against a lurking predator.[1] This often-annoying occurrence represents an evolutionary advantage because it pauses our thought process and primes us for potential danger. It's an interesting example of the many ancient mechanisms that no longer fit the needs of our modern lives, yet still have the potential to control our behaviours. Even at a cellular level, there are evolutionary mechanisms in place that have the power to either increase or slow our rate of ageing. One of the leading experts in this field, Dr David Sinclair, believes that our ancient ancestors were so familiar with 'times of plenty' and 'times of scarcity' that our biology has been primed to recognise and respond to these extremes. He argues that if we are always comfortable, fed or sedentary, our cellular ageing actually increases. Whereas, if we find ways of challenging ourselves or even endure short periods of controlled discomfort, for example undertaking strenuous exercise, our rate of ageing will slow.[2]

If we truly want to be healthier in old age, first we have to go back to basics and engage our primitive brain and biology with something that it will recognise: strength training.

Our ancient instincts and biological impulses are often triggered in modern life and impact on our ability to maintain muscle mass as we age. By using strength training as a form of challenging, yet controlled physical activity, we are using our bodies as they have evolved to be used, forcing us to focus our mind on movement so that we can find the key to a healthy older age.

Standing on stressed shoulders

Irrespective of your achievements in life, if you have reached middle age and are reasonably healthy, you are a winner. You win because the information contained within your biology has got you to this point in history. You represent your ancestral line of kick-ass warriors, hunters, explore, protectors and nurturers who survived when others did not. To a certain extent, we are all standing on the strong shoulders of our ancestors, who have handed down adaptations within our genetic information, biological systems and behavioural traits that help us navigate life. In effect, we have the nervous system of a hunter-gatherer in a modern world.

Without a doubt, our ancient ancestors would be confused by our technologically modern area, but more so by the lack of strength or movement required to survive in today's world. I use the word 'survive' because many of us who make it to older age will be merely surviving, reliant on others for care, rather than thriving as independent, vibrant, older humans. To thrive in older age, we need to have brought our bodies along for the ride by keeping it strong and using it to remain fit and active. However, the challenge is doing this in an environment that has an almost infinite number of ways of triggering our stress response. It is true that we can now expect a comparably longer life, which, for the most part, is free from the physical danger our ancestors faced. That said, the complexity and inactivity of modern living represents a clear and present danger to our long-term strength, due to the subsequent stress that many of us seem to accept as the norm.

Too much stress is not strength's friend

In the previous chapter, I talked briefly about the sympathetic system (fight and flight) and the parasympathetic system (which returns us to a state of calm), the two divisions of the automatic nervous system. This is the network of nerves that controls the day-to-day functioning of our bodies; it is called 'automatic' because it operates without any conscious effort on our part. We are now going to explore in more detail at how the actions of the sympathetic and parasympathetic systems affect our strength. When we experience stress, our sympathetic nervous system is triggered. This means that a broad spectrum of biological responses is set in motion, such as an increase in heart rate and blood pressure, widening of airways, slowing down of digestion, the appearance of goosebumps and heavier sweating. Great! I hear you say, so what's the problem (apart from the sweating and goosebumps)? The problem is that if we are exposed to such responses over the long term, we are at risk of developing hypertension, obesity, insomnia and depression. It's a bit like driving with your foot firmly on the accelerator, when you should be controlling your speed by applying the brake.

Aside from the very real health concerns above, excessive time spent with our sympathetic nervous system in charge also decreases our chances of building and maintaining strength, because we can only do so efficiently when our bodies are in the relaxed parasympathetic state.

But before you decide that the sympathetic nervous system is our enemy, think again. It is what enables us to do challenging physical work, including strength training, whilst also acting to maintain our bodies' ability to function during a training session. Let's not forget that it will also endeavour to protect us should we experience a real threat or emergency. So, although stress is primarily associated with negative experiences, it is a vital element of life and can be a positive stimulating force against which we grow and learn. Anyone who has sat an exam will know just how this looming pressure can negatively affect quality of life. Yet equally familiar is the feeling of elation and achievement at having completed this feat. Likewise, athletes are able to positively harness their stress response and use it to their advantage in physical competition. *Eustress* is a term coined to describe such positive stress experiences, as opposed to *distress*, which refers to the more negative physiological effects of stress that can often overwhelm us. Eustress is a profoundly helpful tool in relation to strength because we can channel it for a productive strength-training session, for example, motivating ourselves with lively music or an inspirational podcast that puts us in a more sympathetic state of arousal. So there really is a balance to be struck in how we perceive and then use this biological legacy.

Happily, there is much that we can do to take more control over our reactions to stress and how we perceive our levels of threat in day-to-day life. Because understanding how modern life influences stress and our chances of long-term strength has never been more important.

Too much of a good thing
The sympathetic state is brought to life in Chops, my spirited Labrador,

who loves nothing better than running and eating. The problem is that if I were to leave Chops to his own devices, he would choose to run (and probably eat) all day if he could, leaving himself exhausted and likely injured. Similarly, as humans we should not spend all day in an excitable state because it leaves us drained and unable to fully recuperate. Physical overtraining causes high levels of cellular inflammation that decrease the quality of our muscles. Similarly, chronic exposure to stressful environments or experiences are the equivalent of overtraining for our hormonal and nervous systems. In everyday life, whether in a work or home setting, prolonged time spent in a sympathetic state increases the prevalence of mental health issues, fatigue and burnout, all of which predispose us to weakness and frailty in old age.

But it is possible to take control of our stress triggers and harness them to work for us. For example, we can navigate from a sympathetic state to a parasympathetic state using simple breathing tools. In physical exercise, this might look like the end of a training session in which you quickly bring your breathing under control to reach a point of relaxation. The same relaxation tools can also be implemented to calm a stress response when at home or work. The more we use these stress-calming strategies in controlled situations, such as relaxing after exercise, the better we become at deploying them in everyday life, for example, when another driver cuts us up on the motorway or we're having a difficult work or personal conversation. The key takeaway here is that it's not just the act of strength training that gets us stronger; it is also the ability to move into a parasympathetic state of relaxation. Improving our capacity to harness and control our responses to life's stresses is vital for our mental wellbeing, as well as our strength and health in older age.

The move less, live longer paradox

Ours is an era in which we live longer but move less than we ever have at any point in history. Mechanisation and modern transport dictate not only that we move less but that when we do move, it is along the pavement in highly predictable straight lines or seated within the metal boxes of cars, trains or planes. For most of us, modern life no longer requires us to move in order to survive. A report from the Institute for the Future predicts that around 85% of the jobs that will exist in 2030 have yet to be invented[3] – which begs the question: will this lead to even less physical activity or strength levels than currently seen? I am sure most of us appreciate the benefits that advancements in technology bring to our day-to-day lives. But I would like to think we can avoid becoming as passive as the humans depicted in the 2008 movie *WALL.E!*, who found it unnecessary to move at all, due to the assistance of their all-encompassing technology.

Only 90 years ago, adults' average heart rate was consistently lower than it is today.[4] This small yet powerful measure of stress is a real-time indicator of how our biology has responded to the changing modern environment, given the direct relationship between heart rate, stress levels and overall health.

The lack of movement in modern working environments suppresses the ancient archetypes of explorer, farmer, warrior and survivor and has an insidious effect upon many health parameters. Although sitting in offices seems to be the efficient and typical way of working in this era, it is none the less disastrous for our mental wellbeing and physical strength.

We should consider trying to find ways of moving more in all aspects of our lives, especially in office settings. I find that walking meetings are a great excuse to move and create a sense of team camaraderie. Standing desks also have their place, but the ideal would be workplaces that provide opportunities and encouragement for exercise during working hours.

But don't worry if this seems unlikely to happen at your place of work. There are still many things you can do to stay active and strong as an individual. Sometimes we just need to be gently reminded of where we came from.

Forgotten archetypes

By now it is clear that the primitive brain is hard-wired for movement. Even if we have never experienced strength training per se, we have evolved by becoming exceedingly good at constant and unpredictable movement, which our primitive brains will recognise and enjoy.

The problem with the sympathetic nervous system is that it is not a good listener. When this system is in charge – when we are scared or angry, during a stressful or a long office workday – our ability to think straight is often compromised.

During my fire service career, fear, pain, anger and terror were emotions that I experienced personally and witnessed in others at countless incidents. It took years of exposure to dangerous events to develop the clarity of thought to make instant life and death decisions. Some experts in emergency decision-making suggest that those of us who must deal with such scenarios over the long term are simultaneously having to deal with their own sympathetic nervous response (no doubt explaining the high levels of mental health issues such as PTSD seen in the fire-first responder communities). The ability of people working in emergency services to successfully deal with a crisis in the moment is in part due to the accumulation of experience by repeated exposure to similar incidents.[5]

What is clear to me from such experiences is the (unsurprising) news that people don't think logically when stressed if they have not been trained to do so. On many occasions during my fire service days, I found myself having conversations with people who were in a state of complete emotional meltdown during an emergency; their ability to communicate and make rational decisions evaporated in the face of their panic. One memorable occasion included being asked to take my fire boots off at the front door by the proud owner of a house whose entire top floor was on fire and threatening to engulf neighbouring houses. On an everyday level, if we are not thinking logically due to excessive stress levels, then we are much less likely to make good choices about our exercise or dietary habits. Simple changes, such as breathing exercises, when you feel overwhelmed will quickly quiet your primitive self, returning the control to the logic of your frontal cortex. Removing yourself to a quiet space and focusing on your lower ribs and tummy pushing outwards as you slowly breathe in and out can be a useful tool in your relaxation toolbox. The simple act of nose-breathing whilst walking can also help bring stress under control, especially if that walk is in nature. If life gets too hectic, I do this daily. The combination of movement and mindfulness helps to clear my mind.

Counter-intuitively, it's not just life pressures or stressful emergencies that can trigger sympathetic over-arousal – lack of activity at home or at work will also influence which part of our autonomic nervous system is in charge and damage our ability to repair and replenish our skeletal muscle. The first step we can take is to remind ourselves that we *can* do challenging things, which, whilst they may seem threatening, will be quickly recognised and accepted by our mind and body. It's hard-wired into us, evolved in response to thousands of generations of activity. You just need to make the smallest of starts to be reminded of what we are here to do.

Trying not to die

As explained, we will avoid any activity that our primitive brains assess as dangerous or foreign. This is a stark reminder that the primary role of the sympathetic nervous system is NOT TO DIE. In the case of strength training, which we know from the introduction, represents a *foreign activity* for the majority of middle-aged men and women (7 and 4% respectively), such poor uptake starts to make sense.

If you have ever been startled by a loud noise that occurred outside your field of vision, you were experiencing another primitive survival mechanism. You may not have noticed at the time, but you would have instantly (and automatically) turned your head towards the source of the noise. In that instant, your primitive brain would have made a decision, determining whether further action was needed to stay safe. We have all experienced this and are familiar with the feeling of a short-lived adrenaline rush that accompanies such situations. This survival reflex (also referred to as the 'hunter's' or 'orientation reflex', first described by physiologist Ivan Sechenov in 1863[6]) is yet another demonstration that our primitive ancestors live on within us.

DAVID VAUX

I think of our primitive nervous system as a silent but surly bodyguard who is on constant lookout for potential threats and ready to step in if danger occurs. Ideally, we do not need our bodyguard to react unless it is an actual emergency, and thankfully, these emergencies are pretty rare for most people day to day.

Getting to grips with strength

A strong grip would have been a key requirement for the survival of our primitive ancestors. On the face of it, it doesn't seem necessary in modern life – but in fact grip continues to be a crucial requirement if we are going to survive and thrive in older age.

I often suggest to strength-training novices that grip strength is a good place to start. Simply put, on a practical level, without a good grip we can't effectively or safely participate in strength training.

How is your handshake? Is it firm or a bit limp? Do you have a family member, as I did, whose Christmas party trick is to crack walnuts with their bare hands? I remember my great-uncle Ted would take immense pleasure in this feat of strength, which to 10-year-old me seemed impossible. Ted was a retired army officer who had also served in the infantry and the army fire service. On retirement, he had stayed highly active, tending to his smallholding in Hythe in Kent and keeping up with his daily exercise regime that had started during World War II. I will never forget his words of advice at the time: that to be a useful human, we need to be 'wiry, athletic and strong'. Uncle Ted certainly was, and when I started my osteopathy practice, I saw that the patients who were in their nineties and still living their best lives, certainly conformed to this archetype. It seems Ted was on to something, and he certainly had a handshake that you would not easily forget.

Many cultures around the world interpret the strength of a person's handshake as an indicator of their vitality and integrity. On a more practical level, do you have a person in your house that you always turn to when a stubborn jar of marmalade needs opening, or are you lucky enough to be that person? Older people with a weak grip are sometimes unable to perform the most basic of tasks, such as holding a plateful of

77

food, and often rely on others to help them. In terms of safety, a strong grip can steady us if we trip, and importantly, allow us grab onto something if we do fall. It is strange then, that we don't often talk about the part grip has to play when working towards a healthy lifestyle. Certainly, in my time as a fire service physical education officer, the grip test was one of the main physical measures that had to be passed to gain entry to fire recruit training school. It is surprisingly rare to find anyone who actively seeks to improve this area, even among those who are strength-training. Unless you know a climber or fighter, it is highly unlikely that anyone in your life is even considering doing so, especially in middle-age. But this is exactly what we need to be doing, and as much as possible, because grip strength in middle age is a powerful predictor of future health.[7] The stronger our grip, the better our chances of older age health.

I like to use the expression 'we are only as strong as our weakest part'. My own weak spot is my lower-back mechanics, which were compromised by injury. For others it might be a knee or an Achilles tendon. But whatever your obvious weakest link is, we all share the modern-day affliction of a weak grip.

A strong grip indicates a person is more active and they are more likely to have created resistance for the muscles of their bodies that have then responded by being stronger. To me it is an indicator that they have been active and will likely continue to be, and consequently stronger in years to come.

This is partly because a strong grip is one of the central mechanisms that send a message to our bodies that we are not ready to age just yet. This starts to make sense when we consider the emphasis that we place on the hands within the somatosensory cortex – the area of the brain that we touched on earlier in the book and will again in the next chapter.

As to how or if a strong grip directly influences our rate of ageing, that remains a mystery. However, we can be confident that an indirect relationship does exist. It is indisputable that a good grip underpins our ability to strength-train and save ourselves from serious injury during a fall, and can subsequently underwrite our chances of an independent life in our old age. For this reason, grip is a key strength that we should endeavour to improve and maintain.

I encourage you in no uncertain terms to 'Get a grip'!

Seeing is believing

A large percentage of the brain's capacity is allocated to sight and movement. This affords us an insight into how *Homo sapiens* survived and went on to successfully colonise and dominate all regions of the world.

We have evolved to prioritise the ability to move; to run, climb, walk, build, fight, hunt and carry. Over time, the ability to be upright with clear fields of view and to use our hands has driven much of human evolution. Remember when I said that the number one goal of our primitive brains is not to die? If our vision is compromised, our primitive brains will act to protect us by slowing us down. We all know that regular eye tests are essential for eye health, but few consider the impact that vision has our strength and posture. Without good strength and flexibility, the ability of our upper back and neck to hold our head in an upright position will be severely compromised.

Sadly, it is all too common to see an older person with a stooped head position, slumped shoulders and sunken ribs that make it impossible for them to stand up straight. This often predisposes them to more difficulties in many everyday movements and increases their chances of pain, inactivity and frailty. Yet within my clinic, I am often met with confusion when I highlight the importance of maintaining good postural habits for our long-term chances of preserving optimal vision and, in turn, strength. I explain that if, like most of us, you have ever suffered from a stiff/sore shoulder (when stressed or sitting still for long periods), it was probably your trapezius muscle – the paired triangular muscle that spans both sides of our shoulders and neck – that is causing the problem. If we experience long-term stress or sit for prolonged periods, this muscle is more likely to increase in tension, which is not only uncomfortable, but also sends a message to the smaller postural muscles, below the trapezius and supporting our spine, that it's 'OK' to weaken. It's a bit like going walking in bad weather, dressed in an outer waterproof jacket (trapezius) and a base layer (deep spinal muscles). If your waterproof jacket is in bad condition, the rain and wind will quickly seep past the outer layer to overwhelm your base layer, compromising its ability to maintain a normal neck and head position.

This long-term loss of function within these smaller postural muscles leads to the slumped postures and slower walking speeds that are so prevalent in the elderly. In relation to how we perceive the world, this will trigger a feedback loop of stress between a poor field of vision and muscle tension.

Given that many people in the modern workplace also sit for eight hours a day hunched over a screen, it is now more crucial than ever that we try to prevent our joints from shortening prematurely and our smaller postural muscles from detraining due to inactivity or static positions. Prolonged sitting in middle age is essentially practice for poor posture in later life. Adding to this problem is the increase in device usage, further encouraging us to move less at home. It seems that slouching over a device is the new norm.

As to the long-term impact of chronic device usage on musculoskeletal health, we will have to wait and see. But in the short term, there is plenty we can do to help ourselves, such as changing our perception of the typical working environment to help decrease the level of stress to which we are exposed. We can also benefit from addressing static working postures by adopting mobility strategies and prioritising our postural strength to minimise muscle detraining. (See Part 2 for the 10 Foundational Movements, in which you will find mobility exercises, paired with strength advice for key areas of the body.)

A balanced life can save us

From an evolutionary perspective, standing upright gave us an advantage that allowed us to move across an environment safely whilst our brains could concentrate on communication, finding food or scanning for other threats. To achieve this safely, we rely on constant feedback from our body sense or (proprioception) and balance. Balance is an element of our daily lives that most take for granted. That is, until we have a problem with it, which, as we know from Chapter One, can be devastating. Balance, like other human functions, is prone to ageing and sensitive to lack of use, meaning that if we don't train our balance, our risk of falling increases. We already know that maintaining the strength of our skeletal muscles also acts to preserve our balance, by improving the function of the nerves that activate them to move. In addition, we know that training for speed and strength, i.e. power exercises, also increases the speed at which our fast-twitch muscle fibres can respond to danger. Doing power exercises means we choose to do an action with the intention to be faster. Training for power basically builds a better pathway for our reflexes to use in an emergency such as a fall.

We save ourselves from falling by scanning our environment for potential trip hazards and relying on constant feedback from our senses to give us a real-time assessment of the types of surfaces we are travelling across (we need our upright posture, good field of vision and strong grip at the ready for this). This everyday mechanism usually works well enough to prevent the vast majority of accidents. But we also rely on the ability of our mind–body connection to rapidly respond in order to avoid falling. Such a scenario usually includes a rapid contraction of our fast-twitch muscle fibres, correcting our foot position from a stumble, or quickly reaching and grabbing onto something. But by far the most amazing reflex triggered in the event of a fall is a rapid tensing of our muscles to form a kind of protective armour around us.

Other reflexes, such as pulling your hand rapidly away when you've touched something hot or sharp occur in an incredible 10–30 milliseconds. As we know, the mind–body connection (nervous system–muscle contraction) benefits from regular strength and power-based training. This is because the nerves that activate our muscles in any strength-related training also get a workout from the activity. They need to be used to remain viable – just like the muscle itself. But we can also train this connection in everyday activities by combining some balance and foot strength into our exercise routines or everyday activities. For suggestions on how to do this, see Chapter 7: *Strength and balance snacks.*

A game of two halves

When I first started to study the human nervous system, I was fascinated to learn that many of the movements we take for granted are actually being controlled by the opposite side of our brains. Meaning that most nerve pathways between our brains and our spinal cords have to physically cross over our mid-lines at some point. The reason for this process, referred to as decussation, remains mysterious and is thought to have happened somewhere along our evolutionary journey.

The game in action

Try visualising yourself as a person with two physical halves. Closing your eyes, picture the right side of your brain, just above your right eye. Now with your mind's eye, draw an imaginary line from the right side of your brain down your neck, across your left shoulder and into your left arm where it finally meets your fingers. Now try closing your eyes and doing the same exercise, only now gently move the fingers of your left hand. Repeat this thought process with the left side of your brain, tracing it down your right shoulder and into your right arm and fingers. Do you feel the connection?

This simple act nicely demonstrates the fact that many of the movements we perform countless times are controlled by the opposite side of the brain. This is an everyday-yet-fascinating mechanism that underpins our ability to move whilst also providing clues to other beneficial health outcomes.

Biological mechanisms, such as decussation, balance and proprioception, are important to strength because without them, our nervous system will put the brakes on again, meaning we will move more slowly and with more caution. But caution is good, right? Well, yes and no. Of course, we should act with caution in certain situations like crossing a road or driving. But we don't always want to be cautious in everyday activities like walking. In such activities, we ideally need to move freely and with confidence.

If we are exposed to pain, fear or change in our patterns of movement for any reason – including lack of motivation to exercise – then we are detraining not only our bodies, but also our brains and consequently our ability to move freely. Our mind–body connection needs to be challenged in order to convince our nervous system that we are not ready to age. Ageing will come to all of us in time, but the simple act of moving confidently and being strong like our ancestors can help us stave off that process for as long as possible.

This does not sound too relevant to strength until we realise our brains are constantly receiving feedback on how we are moving. Remember earlier when I said if we continue to do challenging athletic things our brains will buy into this reality? Conversely, if we sit for too long, the assumption will be that sitting is our norm. If our brains receive the message that we move slowly, without confidence or full bodily range, or with pain and fear, then irrespective of health, we will be guaranteed a downward trajectory well before our time. To prevent this, we need to combine cardio-focused training with strength, as well as regular balance work. The latter can be incorporated into your normal daily routine, with simple exercises like standing on one leg whilst brushing your teeth. Or if this is easy, try closing an eye or alternating the hand you use.

If this sounds like a lot of boring effort, keep reminding yourself of the long and healthy life you will live for just a bit of investment now. Your physical pension will pay off sooner than you think.

Let's get high, naturally!

It is fascinating to me that our bodies will reward us with feeling pleasure when we exercise, due to the hormonal pathways that have been created during our evolution as a species. It's the hormonal equivalent of an encouraging thumbs-up or pat on the back when we participate in feel-good exercise.

Perhaps like me you have had moments of euphoria, inspiration or profound relaxation following your run, something known as a 'runner's high'. This is caused by the endorphin hormones that are released by the brain. The effect might also explain why practitioners of yoga often describe feeling sensations of bliss or experiencing altered states of consciousness following a session. But it's not just runners and yogis who have such pleasurable feelings. In fact, any vigorous exercise can elicit them, including strength training.

It's common for people to report alertness or even excitement during and after strength-focused activities. For those of you have not experienced this (yet), I am not talking about weightlifters screaming and shouting as they lift, but more a feeling of hyper-alertness. Something that I refer to as the *quickening*.

You may have heard this term before, if you have seen the 1986 movie *Highlander*, in which Sean Connery helps Christopher Lambert feel the life force (or quickening) flowing through his body. To be clear, I am not proposing that we try to tap into any external forces, but rather that we relish the release of feel-good hormones, as well as the heightened concentration, physicality and alertness that strength training can bring.

5

Pain, Injury, Fatigue and Strength

'Superhuman effort isn't worth a dam unless it achieves results.'

Ernest Shackleton[1]

When talking to a middle-aged group of people with an interest in making changes to their long-term fitness or wellbeing, I often start by asking for a show of hands for anyone experiencing pain or coping with a niggling injury that has been around for a while. A fair number of hands also go up when I ask if anyone has had a significant injury or illness that has kept them for exercising. For others, their experience of pain will be characterised by long working hours in static positions, which as we know, allow their aching muscles to weaken and become painful over time. Pain in middle age seems to be accepted as the norm, with this association often continuing into later life.

Pain also features prominently within my work in developing exercise resources for those with long-term health conditions or for older cohorts. Simply put, pain and injury are two of the greatest barriers to participation in strength training (or any other exercise): sobering when we consider that a recent systemic review and meta-analysis found that one third to one half of all adults in the UK (just under 28 million people) are affected by chronic pain.[2] This is important because pain and injury are often enough to curtail healthy exercise or activity levels permanently, igniting a feedback loop between pain and loss of strength, often starting in middle age.

Fatigue and burnout are also common features of middle age; we often push our bodies through rearing children, working long hours and consuming a excessive amounts of alcohol to combat the stress, without adequate time spent in rest and recovery. Many people experience long-term chronic fatigue from the sheer demands of everyday life, which is compounded by unwise exercise choices that often prioritise extreme activities, such as high-intensity cardio boot camps, running or spin classes. Pain, injury and fatigue represent the perfect storm for any middle-aged person seeking to stay strong, active and healthy.

In this chapter, we will seek to better understand how our pain system acts; it can often provide protective and beneficial outcomes in the short term, but if we don't respond in the right ways, our pain can become chronic. In learning more about the different types of pain and common preventable injuries of middle age, we will be able to recognise when to push ourselves and when to pause or alter our training. We will also seek to better understand fatigue and the value of good rest and recovery in preventing it. If we learn to listen to our bodies and understand pain, we are setting ourselves up for a successful-long-term strength journey.

Strength as pain relief

It's fascinating that pain can be both useful and harmful in our quest to build older-age strength. We are all familiar with the idea that we can feel pain either quickly or slowly – think of the sharp pain that lets us know a bug is biting us, as opposed to the slow pain in our back when we sit in the same position for too long. However, if pain is present for a long time, such as in an arthritic joint, our nervous system can become oversensitive, causing us to feel more pain more often, and even needlessly. As we know from Chapter 4, our nervous system makes us hard-wired to quickly react to potential harm, as when we pull our hand away from a hot surface or correct a stumble. Less helpfully, our primitive brains will respond to feelings of threat by switching to sympathetic flight-fight mode even when we are not actually in danger. Unfortunately, increased stress levels actually predispose us to feel more pain. This is often exacerbated by our innate human instinct to find the path of least resistance for our bodies in order to avoid further pain. In other words, our brains seek to naturally avoid situations that are painful or uncomfortable. And to a point, this is a great system. However, if we were to avoid anything with an element of challenge, our lives would be much poorer for it (remember when we discussed eustress, the potentially beneficial type of stress, or controlled discomfort that can provide the motivation for us to improve and grow?).

For many of us, pain reduces our motivation to exercise, even when we experience only mild discomfort. A great example of working against our natural instinct to avoid or minimise pain and increase our resilience is the relatively new phenomenon of cold-water exposure made famous by Wim Hoff, which is genuinely quite painful! In my case, my brain tried everything it could to get me out of the water as quickly as possible, within just seconds initially. But with repeated exposure over time, I learned to control my inner voice and increase my pain threshold, with the dawning realisation that I was not actually going to die. After a while I even started to enjoy the sensation, which I found fascinating given the very real experience of pain I had initially.

It makes sense, then, that some people avoid exercise and in particular strength training due to their perception of this very activity being threatening or painful. It is a little-known fact that strength training can actually *decrease* joint pain and is also highly effective in its application to injury prevention, both within elite sports and to those recreational exercisers investing in their long-term health, i.e. you!

The circle of strife

There are many cyclical relationships in nature, including biological and behavioural mechanisms that we often take for granted. An obvious example is the thermoregulation pathway that keeps us at a safe temperature, reacting to our environment to either increase or decrease body heat. There is also the childbirth positive loop, in which the baby's growth stimulates uterine release of oxytocin, the hormone that initiates delivery. It all sounds very 'circle of life', but it is also very relevant to pain and strength when we consider the more negative loops that go on to influence our attitudes towards strength in older age: for example a victim of weight-related bullying in the playground often goes on to have low self-esteem and therefore an increased likelihood of unhealthy eating habits. But I wonder if many of us have ever considered the impact of pain on both our biology and behaviour when it comes to maintaining the health of our skeletal muscle? If we are not careful, it will keep us firmly on a path of immobility and weakness.

As we know, chronic pain affects a large proportion of the UK population and increases with age. Our relationship with pain is one of the mechanisms that works against us in our fight to offset the age-related decrease in skeletal muscle and strength. If we experience pain, from an injury or joint issues, we tend to avoid exercise and movement. As shown in the diagram on the left below, this leads to weakening muscles and yes, you guessed it, increased pain!

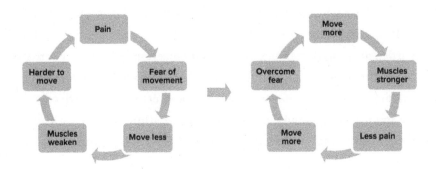

Pain and strength have a relationship that is interrelated in many ways. Excessive pain means you will move far less, and you will feel more pain from joint stiffness due to immobility. You are also likely to feel more pain in a joint that has weaker muscles around it. This is because far from being merely the movers of a joint, our skeletal muscles also act to brace and protect our joints. But in later life, we can only take advantage of this if we have taken the time to develop and maintain these protective muscles – ideally in middle age. Let's return to our maturing vineyard that we have spent years cultivating and maintaining. If we stopped tending to it for a few years, it would limp on and produce some wine, but it would be of poor vintage.

Our joints are only as good as the strength of the surrounding muscles. Often in clinic I see decreases in long-term pain, even in an arthritic joint, if the person manages to strengthen the muscle around it. It is for the same reason that surgeons will encourage people expecting joint replacement surgery to lose weight and exercise as much as possible. Firstly, so that they are less likely to suffer any negative effects from the anaesthetic, but mainly because they will have the best chance of a quick recovery if they have strong muscles. Whilst there are some incredible medical advancements in joint surgery, such as clothing with embedded technology that can assess and assist movement, for the time being we need to rely on good old-fashioned muscle to power the movement in our joints.

My own journey out of the show-stopping pain I acquired in the fire service started with the realisation that, to a point, I was always going to live with pain. I knew I had a decision to make. I could either spend the rest of my life letting pain dictate my every move – slowly becoming weaker, inactive and unhealthy. Or I could choose to listen to my body and combat pain to stay strong, active and healthy. Happily, the latter choice has led to decreased pain, improved health and overall enjoyment of life. This is possible for all who live with pain, but only once you are able to accept and reframe the meaning of it.

Cornered by pain

If left unchecked, pain can become the most dominant factor in your life and come to define who you feel you are. If you have ever been cornered at a party by a relative who doesn't let you get a word in edgeways, you have no option but to listen. Our interactions with pain can be strikingly similar, meaning, if you have become trapped by inactivity, your experience of pain becomes more intense, even overwhelming. However, if you choose to break away from that corner to move, dance, laugh and listen to the music, even though the relative will still be talking, you will have broken the cycle; the drone will become background noise and will not dominate your thoughts. You will have regained control back of your life, breaking the pattern of inactivity. In a nutshell, pain is more intense if we allow it to make us inactive.

I have had more than my fair share of pain. But you might be surprised to hear that educating myself on this subject has been as essential as movement or strength training on my road to recovery. There are many types of pain and reasons for its appearance. But did you know that it's not only movement-based strategies but also our intellectual effort that help decrease pain? Not surprisingly, there is a great deal of research on understanding pain; its purpose, when it is useful, when it goes wrong, and how to think about it. In their seminal work *Understanding Pain*, David Butler and Lorimer Mosley explain that pain, far from being an unusual occurrence, is actually quite normal.[3]. They demonstrate how our thoughts alone can directly influence its impact on our lives.

So pain is all in our heads after all, right?

Well, yes and no. It is true that the majority of those who have experienced long-term pain will at some point be told dismissively, 'it's all in your head'. Especially, as is often the case, if an X-ray or MRI fails to show any reason for their symptoms. (It is not uncommon for an MRI of a lower back to reveal no obvious explanation for very real back pain.)

We sense pain via a complex system of neurons that cover our entire body. The body's millions of pain sensors are attached to nerves that converge in our spines and then travel to our brains. The pain signal that may have originated in the toe you have just stubbed – or the thumb you have just accidentally hit with a hammer – passes through several systems that literally decide if this signal is worthy of being forwarded towards our brains (working as a *pain gateway* of sorts). So, it is indeed true that pain is felt in the head, but only because our head houses our brain. Although interestingly, our brain tissue does not actually contain pain receptors.

A nice way of thinking about our pain system is to compare it to a sports team, with medical staff and a manager. The sports team are your pain sensors/nerves that are ready to respond to any kind of injury, such as inflammation, poor blood flow or low oxygen, microdamage, extremes of temperature, illness or other insults to your body. The sports team are ready to sense any such occurrence at any time. The medical staff are your spinal cord, receiving and filtering the incoming messages from your pain sensors (sports team). The medical team observe from the pitch side (as I have done on countless occasions), responding to an injured player (pain signal) by assessing the seriousness of the injury and deciding whether to escalate it to the manager (your brain). Often the medical team (spinal cord) will assess the signal as minor and not worthy of the manager's (brain's) attention.

The 'medical teams' that act as filters or gateways for pain signals in our own bodies are housed in areas of our spinal cords known as pain gates. Which, far from being merely reactive to pain, can actually be utilised to reduce pain through some very simple strategies.

Closing your pain gate

If you ever fell over as a child, did you run to a nearby parent, teacher or relative, who would literally rub the injured area and magically make your pain disappear? If so, sadly this was not actual magic, but one of your pain gates at work within the spinal cord, helping to decrease or block the amount of pain able to make it up to the brain. Grabbing or rubbing an injured area results in the sensors responsible for touch in that area sending their own signal to the spinal cord. This new signal works to close the pain gate and decrease the pain. The Pain Gate Theory was first described by academics Ronald Melzack and Patrick Wall in 1965,[4] who explained the many steps it takes for the brain to receive information about an area of your body. But it also illustrates that our spinal cord is not merely dealing with pain signals but are also witness to and influenced by many aspects of our lives.

For instance, one of the other factors that influences our pain gate is our state of mind or mood. One of the reasons we experience more pain when depressed, anxious or tired is that these states are all known to influence the pain gate. But we don't even need to be in those states to experience more pain. In relation to our postures, long-term physical tension, as seen in immobile working positions, will mean that many of our muscles are switched on all the time. In time, the physical tension caused by such postures increases our general level of discomfort and in turn stress, meaning that not only will the muscle affected not relax, but the nervous system will presume that the body is under some level of duress. Which it is! Unfortunately, this negative loop only serves to open the pain gate and make us more prone to higher levels of pain reaching our brains. And as we also know, chronic tension in muscles weakens them over time.

Something that helps all kinds of pain is moving more and not letting your home or working life be defined by lack of movement. We can all find ways of being less static and more fluid in the ways we use our bodies. Movement is literally the pain medicine we need, and our muscles are the big spoon we use to take it. Which is another reason to keep them strong!

Be like water

Do not get set into one shape or form, adapt it and build your own, be like water.' This quote is associated with the legendary filmmaker and martial artist Bruce Lee. Although he said it in the context of martial arts, it is just as relevant to pain.

On page 60, I said that if we spend a long time sitting, our brains will in time accept this as who we are and we will adapt to become very good at it. Far from being just a state of mind, prolonged sitting has a very real effect on our nervous system, because as we have just learned, low physical activity will also open the pain gate. Conversely, movement that includes exercise and strength training can prevent your pain system from being oversensitive. The challenge here is that for anyone who has experience of long-term pain (me included), the last thing they want to do is move. It's not an easy thing to do, but we must try to overcome the very understandable hesitancy to move when in pain. The key is to find a way of moving without triggering a pain response. This can vary greatly depending on the person, their lifestyle, and the cause of the pain.

The starting point on my own journey was to find ways of moving my body in water, and the same has been true of many of my patients. The simple act of unweighting our bodies in water can be a great way of sending 'movement messages' up the spine – around the pain gate, which has been wedged open by previous pain – so that they reach the brain without the accompanying pain messaging. Over time, such movement starts to help close the pain gate and improve the overall level of pain that we are experiencing.

My nuisance neighbour still arrives at my front door from time to time. Thankfully, though, I can avoid a drawn-out conversation and have learned to quickly quiet them with the exercise and movement that works for me and allows me to close the door!

Painful lessons

If you have ever twisted an ankle and then immediately tried to stand up, you will have quickly realised that you no longer have control over your body. Try as you may, you just can't walk or even contract the muscles needed to hobble and limp to the front door. What is happening here is that your very clever fail-safe system has kicked in to stop you doing any further damage to your ankle. In this first phase of an injury, pain and motor neurons form a close relationship in which the former tells the latter to stop that body part from moving. If this is not a serious injury, this relationship fades until one day – and often unexpectedly – you can move again. However, in a more serious injury, this can go on for longer than is actually needed, and in some cases even when the injury is long healed, you are unable to fully activate that muscle.

Similarly, the phenomenon of phantom pain can leave amputees continuing to experience real pain from a limb that is no longer there.[5] My own injury was much less dramatic: I experienced multiple spinal disc prolapses at the same time (a condition whereby inner discal gel escapes from the disc). The trouble is that if the gel presses on a nerve it can cause long-term changes. As a result of my injury, I have an oversensitivity in my spine that will react to even a slight muscle strain in the region of my back that was originally damaged. This is due to the sciatic nerve, spinal cord and brain all being bombarded with pain signals, albeit 20 years ago. Subsequently, the pain gate for my original spinal injury now has a 'hair trigger', meaning it is more sensitive than in someone who has not experienced such an injury.

The lesson here is that although an original biological injury may have long since healed, our nerves, spinal cords and brains can take far longer to return to normal. It's a bit like a floodgate being opened, turning a once tranquil stream into a raging torrent. In time, the flood will subside, but the stream is unlikely to ever return to its original state, and the water is unlikely to take its previous path.

However, if you had a long-term injury that sometimes triggers pain for no particular reason, please rest assured: there is always a strategy that will help you quickly put your phantom back to sleep.

Finding ways of moving without discomfort, when newly injured or when enduring chronic pain, is the bedrock on which much of my pain management approach sits. Because, as outlined in Chapter 4, our primitive brains will interpret pain-free movement as a sign that all is well, thereby minimising our reaction to any injury and ensuring an optimal recovery.

Injury can happen to anyone, and when it does, the smart response is to back off from the activity that caused it, whilst continuing to move, albeit in different ways. As mentioned above, utilising a pool, if possible, is usually an effective starting point, as is removing any external loading (such as weights or other equipment) from your routine. Don't think of this as a backward step, but rather a side-step that cleverly decreases the intensity and time you are exposed to pain.

Gain and pain

If we expect something to hurt, it is probably going to. Actually, it is certain to. This is because raised stress levels are guaranteed to rachet up our entire pain system, and in pain, context is king. If you've ever watched a child fall over and graze their knee or bump their head, you will be familiar with the calm before the storm, when the child will look up for a social cue from the parent about how to respond. If you show horror, so will the child, even in the case of a minor graze. Conversely, if your response is calm, then it's likely the child will show the same response, enabling them to gain control of their pain system. If this sounds straightforward, be warned that this system can be equally dramatic in both directions. To explain this, it might be helpful to describe one of the more famous images that most students studying pain management will be familiar with, involving the case of a worker who stood on a 6-inch nail. The nail in question went straight through the worker's protective footwear, leaving the point of the nail protruding vertically up through the upper surface of this boot. Reports from the medical staff on duty on that day state that the paramedics had to administer pain relief just to transport him to the hospital. The story then goes that when the boot was cut away, the nail was found not to have injured the victim at all. Instead, rather miraculously, it had passed through a gap between his toes!

I am certainly not judging this individual who has become famous, albeit anonymously, in medical circles. In fact, it nicely demonstrates that fear and feelings of threat are impactful enough by themselves to generate real pain.

I am not suggesting that by remaining strong we can avoid standing on a nail; rather, that by remaining strong, thereby retaining our emotional confidence in our physical ability, we are more likely to minimise the impact of pain should it come calling.

Strengthening our braking system will protect us

When was the last time you went for a hike in the hills? If, like me, you enjoy getting into high and wild places, have you also noticed that going downhill often hurts more than going up? Unless you are a mountaineer, anyone who has come downstairs the day after a long run will also be familiar with the pain that often surprises us when navigating a staircase of steep steps. This common experience is down to the fact that it is our knees that must take the strain in most of our exercise choices.

The knee is prone to many injuries (such as the classic runner knee) and traumatic damages to one of its many ligaments are commonly caused by dynamic activities such as football, tennis, running or skiing. But in normal day-to-day life, our knees tend to hurt when we are going downhill because when we do so the load on them is around 3.5 times our actual weight. Meaning, if you weigh 100kg, your knee will be dealing with a 350kg load. All of this sounds scary, but luckily our knees are usually stable due to the ligaments around them and the fact that the rear of the kneecap has the thickest amount of cartilage seen anywhere in the body.

Aside from injury, the main reason for knee pain, especially when walking downhill, is that most of us have not trained to be strong in this movement. What I mean by this is that we value the ability to stand up in life and consequently we get strong in the shortening contraction of the front thigh muscles of this movement. But it is in fact the lengthening phase that, if weak, causes us to have increased knee pain. Weakness in this movement means that the ligaments and cartilage must deal with more of the load. We fall into the trap of pressing our foot hard on the accelerator pedal again, realising too late that we also need to be good at slowing down. It is within our braking system that our long-term safety resides. It isn't our ability to run fast that will protect us, but our ability to slow down rapidly and safely.[6]

We need to work on our braking system to maximise our long-term health, minimising injury and whilst also decreasing the load across our joints. We can all do this by lengthening our muscles under tension in our strength-training routines, which we will explore in Part 2. This can be as easy as standing up to the count of '1-2', then slowly letting your thigh muscles lengthen whilst slowly sitting to the count of '3-4-5-6'.

This simple approach can be applied to the majority of the Foundational 10 movements we want to get stronger in and helps us to reduce the risk of injury and putting too much pressure on our joints. I will explain when to incorporated this type of training in Chapter 7. It will be the only time that focusing on the *negative* is actually really good for us!

Pain and overtraining

Let's be honest, most of us have overdone exercise at some point in our lives. Perhaps we have become really invested in a particular sport, such as running, cycling, tennis, swimming or weight training, that has become all-encompassing. If any of this sounds familiar, you might be interested to know that you may have already passed the point at which you can continue to improve your performance. What I am getting at is that there is a threshold we pass of *decreasing returns* when we fall into the trap of overtraining.

As we touched on earlier, over-training will often negatively influence our fatigue levels, whilst also leading to cellular inflammation within our muscles and connective tissues. In addition, our muscles, ligaments, fascia, and tendons will all eventually suffer if loading is repeated without ample recovery time, sufficient nutrition, sleep and hydration. The subsequent cumulative microtrauma may eventually progress to poor performance and tight, aching or injured muscles. Less dramatically, this microtrauma can manifest in the long term as inflammation of a tendon, such as Achilles tendonitis or similar injuries such as a tennis or golfer elbow. The unifying element across all training injuries is the experience of some form of pain that crops up during or after exercise, or worse – in everyday life when merely walking around the house.

The good news is that such outcomes can be almost entirely

prevented if we take heed of even a minor pain, which in training can often be a warning sign of a more serious injury to come if we continue to exercise in the same way. When I consult with middle-aged clients who are focused on a particularly intense way of getting fit or strong, it is often a hard sell to suggest some variation or reduction in their training. But it is from variation that useful adaptation springs, and the combination of variation plus adequate recuperation is often enough to prevent pain ever rearing its head.

However, the truth is that we can't prevent all pain. Pain in middle age is commonplace and the majority of us will be well accustomed to managing an old injury. Paradoxically, pain is not just a sign of injury or overtraining. It can also be a barometer of helpful physical loading against which our bodies can become stronger. The trick is in becoming fluent in the different dialects of pain.

Body talk: leaning into pain

First and foremost, we need to place our bodies in challenging yet controlled circumstances to improve our strength, cardiovascular efficiency, balance and flexibility over the long term. But what if regular discomfort, albeit in a controlled dose, also had the potential to reduce our cellular rate of ageing? In his 2019 book, *Lifespan*, Dr David Sinclair suggests that participating in controlled discomfort of some kind will help to slow our rate of cellular ageing,[7] whilst being too comfortable or inactive – both physically and intellectually – may serve to accelerate it.

Consistent and progressive strength training is one of the activities we can manipulate to mimic discomfort or challenge, in a controlled and (dare I say) enjoyable way. The idea is not to push our bodies harder into old age. In middle age – despite what we sometimes like to tell ourselves – it is impossible to sustain the energy levels and strength we had as a teenager. What we can exploit, however, is the experience, maturity and discipline that we did not have as teenagers. In the long game of achieving older-age strength, it is consistency and quality that counts, not intensity and quantity. We need to engage in activity that is challenging enough to stimulate improvements in our strength, without getting injured, whilst still sending the message to our deep biology that we are not yet ready to age. And the key to this is understanding that our bodies are talking to us all the time via the language of pain – we just need to learn how to listen.

Embracing the burn

Strength training often causes us to feel a burning pain in the muscles as they are working hard. This can occasionally be intense but is usually short-lived and often disappears completely in between repetitions of an exercise.

The 'burn' can also be a useful tool in ensuring that you are correctly targeting the areas you want to strengthen. For example, if you are trying to strengthen the muscles of your thighs, yet the burning is more focused on your lower-back muscles, then you need to readjust your form or try another exercise until you feel the muscles working in the targeted area. In this regard, it is true that the burn, although to be avoided in the extreme, can serve to confirm we are strengthening the intended area. I would also add that the type of strength training I advocate minimises this experience, as it is more associated with body-building practices. But feeling a mild burn is perfectly fine!

Understanding post workout soreness

The other type of pain that most of us experience around exercise is the one that crops up a day or so after a workout. In serious cases, this can signify an actual injury (especially the week after the parents' sports day!), but more often than not it's something else. Delayed-onset muscle soreness or DOMS is another common experience for anyone who has participated in any challenging or unaccustomed activity. This is because the activity challenged your muscles in ways that they are not used to. In my case, when I played tennis for the first time in 25 years, my glutes or 'rear end' muscles felt that they were on fire for a week. When we load a muscle, it adapts to this stimulation by creating microtrauma in the muscle fibres, causing localised inflammation. In my case, because I hadn't moved in the way tennis requires for years, I overloaded those particular muscles. Strength training causes a similar overloading, albeit in a more controlled way, also leading to the same localised adaptations and in some cases delayed muscle soreness, which is felt following eccentric exercise (lengthening of our muscle under load) or after more dynamic activity, such as running or sprinting.

Far from fearing DOMS, I encourage people to utilise it as a form of self-regulation, a barometer indicating how hard we should or should not be working out. The reality is that it's not necessary to feel muscle soreness following strength training for it to be effective and it is perfectly possible to get stronger and never experience any muscle soreness at all. In fact, it is a good idea, especially in middle age not to push yourself so hard that you risk excessive post workout pain, because as we now know, pain from any source is a serious barrier to exercise.

If you push yourself too hard, DOMS can stop you from training for long periods of time, so you actually end up weaker, which is ironic given the effort you clearly gave to the guilty session. The takeaway here is to train for functional strength around the key joints of your body., to maintain their main direction of movement and also to protect your posture. Simply blasting our biceps to get them as big as possible (as with body building) will not maintain our essential ability to be strong in a pulling movement (such as pulling yourself up from the floor). It is also much more likely that you will experience high levels of DOMS, restricting your ability to train or indeed move effectively in normal life.

So, whilst muscle soreness is not a given to see improvements in strength, it is highly likely you will experience it if you are just starting to explore strength training. However, as we grow more accustomed to strength training, we also gain knowledge on how our bodies respond and how much DOMS to expect. I tend to advise strength training novices to only train a body area if they are on a 1–2 out of 10 in terms of DOMS, meaning they would have a vague awareness of mild aching in the body part in question. If you are more aware of soreness in that area after your warm-up, then keep it a very light session. This may seem simple, however, there are many factors that can throw us a curveball when it comes to our responses to training in middle age.

We have to be realistic that what was a 1 or 2 for muscle soreness last week might be a shocking 5–6 out of 10 the following week, having completed the exact same routine. This often-mysterious occurrence in middle age is in fact completely dependent on what else is going on in our lives before, during and after we train. If we do not sleep, hydrate, refuel, mobilise and relax as well as we did the previous week, our recovery from strength training will also be different. Therefore, we need to learn to interpret how our bodies feel when we have got things wrong, whilst also understanding the feel of when things have gone well. What I mean by this is that given enough time, our bodies will adapt and get stronger. So, one day you will realise that the routine and weight you're using has not changed, but you have not had DOMS for a month or so. In fact, you might also be beginning to feel that the exercise has become easier. This is a real time example of your improving strength because what previously overloaded your muscles no longer does – you have become stronger. This is the time to increase the challenge or difficulty of what you are doing. But be warned, DOMS is likely to make an appearance again if you are not mindful of your body's ability to exercise and recover.

Training when tired makes us weaker

One of the things that defines us as humans is that we can achieve the most incredible feats, even when they initially seem out of reach. This is why finding different ways of challenging ourselves is so good for us, such as taking up a new activity or learning a language. Where this can go astray, however, is when we push ourselves when we actually need to rest, as so often happens when all the hustle and bustle of everyday life seems to demand our full attention. We are talking about one of the most important skills we need to build for healthy older age: the ability to regulate when or how hard we train. Fatigue levels, like muscle soreness, can be used as a useful barometer of *when* to train.

Yes, we can train when we are tired, and many of us try to push through to complete our fitness routines. But the reality is that if we keep ignoring fatigue, then we are unlikely to make any strength or fitness improvements. Worse still, we are risking our ability to be stronger in older age.

Developing this deep knowledge of what our bodies are trying to tell us can take time but is perfectly possible for all of us. Our bodies have incredible wisdom waiting to be accessed.

Just as DOMS is a sign the muscle is not fully recovered, fatigue is a sign that our nervous system has yet to recuperate.

Perhaps you pushed too hard in the previous session and have not slept well? Perhaps there is just too much going on in your life and you arrive at your training session already tired out? Given we are also training the nervous system in strength training, fatigue should be viewed as useful feedback, not just within our exercise routines but also our general lives. We must be mindful and respectful of fatigue in middle age because it is during this stage that we are often at the very edge of our capacity in life. What I mean by this is that any exercise, including strength training, must co-exist with other life stresses, such as work and domestic responsibilities. Because if we overextend ourselves in one aspect of our lives, all others suffer. If we are not careful, we can often tip over into the chronic fatigue and burnout that is so prevalent during this life stage.

Understanding our normal energy levels, how we recover from exercise, and how fatigue can build up will greatly improve our prospects of older-age strength. Because in middle age, not burning out is as important as not getting injured. A simple way of objectively measuring whether you should exercise is knowing what your normal resting heart rate is on waking. If higher than normal, it's highly likely that you are not recovered or adequately rested and therefore it's not a good day to push yourself too hard.

If this is the case, it's a good idea to rest, especially if this increased heart rate is accompanied by feeling fatigued. I always recommend a less challenging version of the workout you may have planned with more emphasis on stretching and relaxation. By tapping into the wisdom of our bodies, they will be able to look after us for longer.

The key message here is that we do not want to let middle age hijack our chances of older-age strength by overexercising ourselves into burnout. In fact, I would reiterate that this is the time in life to rethink our relationship with exercise, as I and many of my patients have successfully done. Because although we can all agree that it was fun to charge around in our cars (or in my case fire engine) at high speed and in low gears during our younger years, this is no longer the most efficient way of getting to our destination safely. In reality, we need to ease into economy mode, switch on cruise control and enjoy a smoother ride. As a result, we will arrive at a stronger older age with more fuel in the tank and with more of our original parts intact.

Staying strong with an injury

It's important to point out that pain from DOMS is different from injury pain. OK, technically DOMS is a form of short-lived and self-inflicted injury (or microdamage to our muscles). But the key difference is that it usually occurs after a controlled exercise session and is a temporary condition. Also, when kept to low levels, DOMS is a side effect of us getting stronger and more able to remain active in life. On the other end of the spectrum, we have ballistic injuries, such as those that occur on falling, tripping or overtraining, which can cause muscle tears, joint strains, stress fractures, tendonitis or ligament injuries. These are not controlled and are going to make us weaker and less mobile.

When injured or having developed something like a repetitive strain injury, we need to stop doing the activity that caused it. After all, Albert Einstein purportedly said: 'The definition of insanity is doing the same thing over and over and expecting different results.' Students of quantum mechanics might now disagree with this statement, but in the field of injury prevention it still rings true. Which is why we would ideally find different ways of keeping fit, strong, and active even with pain or injury.

If you are unlucky enough to find yourself injured on one side, such as in one ankle, knee or shoulder, did you know that you can guard against muscle loss in that region by working on the uninjured side? In this extraordinary process, our nervous system will work to maintain our 'symmetrical system' at all costs, meaning it will do all it can to help us recover movement as quickly as possible. It seems to have a fail-safe method specifically for a one-sided injury. So even if an injured person has a joint they cannot use, if they train the uninjured side, there will be a significant 'crossover effect' that can go a long way to protecting against the worst harms of muscle loss caused by immobility. In essence, if your left knee – or any other joint – is injured, if you continue to strengthen your right knee, it will also benefit the left.

If you are still able to get active despite an injury, perhaps try walking in a pool and gently mobilising as a starting point. Or use a local gym if they have a machine that allows you to move without overloading a particular injured body part.

If all else fails and you can't find a way to move without pain, the bottom line is that the starting point is always in our minds, getting used to visualising pain-free movement in the early stages of being injured. Because if it's good enough for the world's best athletes, it's certainly good enough for a middle-aged strength enthusiast. And the sooner we use such tools, the sooner we will be back to the activities we enjoy and more importantly, the long and healthy older age that awaits us.

The injury dividend

When working with athletes or keep-fit fanatics who are injured, I try to reframe injury as an opportunity. This understandably sounds like a load of rubbish, especially if you partly define yourself by the exercise or activity you enjoy. Unfortunately, you must respect the process of injury and recovery because it does not care if you want to go for a run or play tennis next week. In fact, if you disrespect the process, it will teach you a painful lesson in humility – sometimes an important one for many busy middle-aged men and women reevaluating their life-stage. An injury is often your body's last resort in getting your attention if you have ignored the need to rest, hydrate, stretch, strengthen, or moderate your training. Remember, we need to give ourselves permission to be middle-aged. Part of which should be focused on being able to continuously show up to training for the next 30 years and to be confident enough in ourselves to back off from a session if we feel 'off' for any reason. We need to live to fight and train another day. Injury presents an opportunity to try a different sport or activity that doesn't aggravate our condition, and also invites us to pause and reflect on our goals.

The good news is that one of the biggest clichés in rehabilitation is true: 'it is possible to come back stronger, faster and better following an injury'. There are many inspirational and feel-good stories in sport in which a person overcomes an injury and makes a triumphant comeback. On an everyday level, if we are respectful of what our bodies are trying to tell us, we can return from injury more quickly and even prevent the vast majority of injuries from happening in the first place.

Even if you are not destined to return to what you could previously do following an injury, you can still focus on recovering to your fullest potential, finding other methods of staying active, which far from being a chore might allow you to grow in ways that the old you could never have imagined. Because if you make your comeback and train smarter in the long term, the injury that you experienced could be viewed as a gift. In my case, I know it was.

The great gamble

How many of us who are physically active recognise the mindset of hoping not to get injured, but don't actually do much, if anything, to prevent it? How many of us in middle age have acquired a pattern of exercise from youth and just don't think about injury at all? Isn't it true that what we are secretly saying to ourselves is: 'I am going to train until I am injured – and only then will I stop'? What we are doing is putting our trust in chance and gambling with our bodies in a very high-risk game. We need to be focused on the next 30 years and not the next 30 minutes of strength training.

Every one of us has, at some point, pushed through feeling fatigued or having a niggly pain from a tendon or ligament injury, to do exercise. Unhelpfully for midlifers, many times in the past we have probably got away with it. But as we age, the chance of avoiding injury decreases significantly.

What we should realise is that the middle-aged person needs to win the marathon not the sprint. It's like the old fable of The Tortoise and the Hare; in midlife we definitely want to be the tortoise – which more helpfully for this agegroup, also live significantly longer!

If we don't moderate our often-well-intentioned motivation to 'go hard or go home', we are predisposing ourselves to burnout, injury and increased strength loss over the long term, and setting up a perfect storm for frailty in older age. I do not judge anyone who struggles with this new way of thinking as I was the same, until I was injured. In fairness, I suffered an occupational injury that stopped any training for years. However, with the benefit of hindsight, I feel it was inevitable that the high volume of training I was engaged in would have eventually led me down the path of burnout and injury. In many ways, the injury I sustained was an opportunity to reset my entire outlook on exercise and what my long-term goals should be.

What I have learned from my own experience and from working with some of the most athletic humans on the planet is this: if we are chronically fatigued, overtrained or underrecovered, we are at increased risk of poor health levels in older age. Conversely, and as we know from earlier chapters, inactivity increases the likelihood of chronic pain, injury, frailty, ill health and loss of independence in older age. At either end of the exercise spectrum lies often unmanageable pain and the subsequent increased risk of weakness in older age.

Thankfully, people at both ends of the activity spectrum, can be helped with a 'next 30 years' mindset to strength training, finding challenging, controlled and smart ways of remaining strong, whilst equally valuing rest and recuperation.

We're all in this together

Professional and international sports teams are often shown how to run faster with drills and techniques developed to achieve better performance in the short term. The risk here is that any short-term increase in performance comes with an increase in the forces that the body must deal with, which often results in a build-up of damage in the muscles and connective tissues. The problem is that although a person may have been shown how to run faster, throw further or lift heavier via technique coaching, the muscles and connective tissue have not had sufficient time to adapt. In addition, the nervous system will not have had the time to develop adequate control, which also predisposes the person to increased risk of injury.

This is important because we are all at risk of injury if we go too hard in the first phases of a new sport or activity, such as taking up strength training in midlife. We need to be patient when learning anything from scratch, especially if, like me, you are in any way competitive.

The risk of injury when participating in something new or trying different techniques is very real in professional sports, especially within dynamic team games. When giving conditioning advice to an international sports team with a history of high injury rates, I developed a 3-step programme, which only allowed progression to higher volumes of stress on the body (the final stage replicated game play) after players had mastered the movements in stages 1 and 2. The time spent building musculoskeletal resilience and nervous system control was an investment not only in performance but also in improving the ability to safely deal with increasing physical demands that they encountered. This approach led to significant decreases in non-contact injury that had, until then, blighted squad performance during long tournaments.

It is the same for a person who has little to no history of strength training, in that they too will need longer in the initial strength phases of their programme to prepare for the new forces or demands on their bones, joints, ligaments, tendons, fascia, muscles and nervous system (see Chapter 6: Mimimal Loading Programme). By investing the time at the beginning of your journey, you will end up avoiding the vast majority of injuries from fitness training and indeed normal life. You will have upgraded the strength of your entire system, not just your muscles. Rather like a well-thought-out pension fund, your older-age body will benefit from this wise strength investment and even better, you'll have the energy to see out the rest of your life in glory.

When starting strength training with older-age health as our goal, the reward is to finish strongly. Therefore, our focus should be fixed on the far horizon, not short-term gratification. We should be ready to recognise the signs of injury or fatigue, using our life experience to do so. Even a minor injury has the potential to become something bigger and change the trajectory of our lives. Maintaining our ability to consistently strength train over the long-term is brutally simple: listen to what your body is telling you, know when to train and when to rest, understand pain and don't ignore injury or fatigue.

In doing so you will be well set to begin your march towards later-life health and being faster, more energetic and stronger.

Part 2

6

Understanding Your Strength Starting Point

'No great thing is created suddenly, any more
than a bunch of grapes or a fig. If you tell me that
you desire a fig, I answer you that there must be time.
Let it first blossom, then bear fruit, then ripen.'

Epictetus

There are countless quotes from antiquity that nicely capture the journey towards strength, as the philosopher Epictetus does above. Or perhaps some of you might have come across the name of Milo of Croton from even further back in history. Milo lived in the fifth century BC, and his feats of strength have become the stuff of legend. By all accounts he dominated the wrestling events of the ancient Olympics for decades. Milo is also one of the first names to be associated with the principle of slowly increasing the difficulty of exercise to improve physical performance, otherwise known as 'progressive overload'. The story goes that Milo trained by lifting and carrying a young calf up a hill. As the calf grew larger and heavier, Milo continued to lift and carry the animal, slowly and steadily building his strength over time. Although the practicality of this method seems dubious, it does nicely demonstrate that even in ancient times, people understood the basic principles of progressively adding difficulty to strength training. These days 'calf' training means something different, but the underlying method is much the same!

What this example also shows is that, in the highly digitised era we live in, we often lose sight of the fact that there is a great deal of wisdom to be found within our ancient cultures and indeed within our own bodies. In Chapter 4, we explored how our bodies will literally reward us in the short term with feel-good hormones when we take the right exercise and make us experience fatigue or pain when we over- or underexercise. In blue zones around the world, the elderly population are often as strong, athletic and independent as many younger members of their communities. Even a cursory look at the daily routines of these strong humans will reveal habitual behaviours and ingrained wisdom around exercise, diet, rest, happiness, self-agency and community. Put simply, strength has become a part of life for them. For example, in Okinawa, Japan, the tradition of eating meals and resting on the floor means getting up and down from squatting or sitting cross-legged many times a day, naturally building lower-body strength and balance. This deep-rooted behaviour undoubtedly contributes to protection from frailty and falls in later life and is partly the reason why Okinawans have some of the longest and healthiest lifespans on the planet.

However, habits that belong to other cultures can be difficult or impractical for us to adopt in the West. To make things even more complicated, an almost infinite number of routes to getting fitter or stronger are promoted to us on the news and social media on a daily basis. It can be confusing, and what works for one person almost certainly will not work for all.

The truth is that the unifying ingredients of any strength success story are *always* consistency – finding easy ways to add strength building into your everyday routine – and self-regulation – doing the right amount at the right time.

In this chapter, we will discuss what we can and cannot control in terms of our innate biological potential for strength, whilst getting to grips with our own individual starting points towards a stronger future. Now we know the WHY, it's time to discuss the HOW.

Reimagining your personal best

If we are honest with ourselves, most of us wouldn't choose to grind out a hard exercise session every day, unless we are young and full of energy or working in the military or emergency services, perhaps. If you believe this is sustainable in middle age, you are setting out on your strength journey with unrealistic expectations and failure will surely follow. It is also not realistic to expect to perform as well or indeed better than the last training session every time. So go easy on yourself. Because, as seen in Chapter 5, a whole host of outside influences affect how well we can recover from our last training session. And once we hit middle age, the term *personal best* takes on a completely different meaning. Your personal best should now be structured around *consistency* of strength training with a view to delivering *your best life*. Not over weeks or months, but instead framed in the context of the next 30 years. We are all going to have times when we are injured, ill, pulled away to care for a child or older relative, or focused on an important work deadline. However, the beauty of the long view on strength is that if we engage in regular training from middle to old age, then we cannot fail to have a strong and robust life. Like eating healthily, it is something we need to do *most* of the time, to future-proof our bodies successfully.

Find your rhythm

There are times in middle age when everything seems to conspire against us and the thought of any time to ourselves is but a dream. As we know, middle age is the key life stage in which our future chances of strength and in turn health are often decided. Alongside all the noticeable physiological changes going on in our bodies, we also have to contend with events that are outside our control. It is no surprise that injury or illness can derail your exercise, but have you considered the fallout of someone else in your life becoming injured? It has a knock-on effect on you, filling up free time with caring responsibilities for the injured or ill party. I mention this because, along with pain and fear, life events that in some way change the rhythm of life can have a long-lasting impact on our older-age strength. Consider the couple in which one becomes infirm and the other then devotes themselves to looking after them, often at the cost of their own health. Or the person who retires and gradually stops exercising due to ageist narratives. Or even moving house or changing jobs, which can often curtail any thoughts of exercise for long periods of time.

I have written this book to remind people that, far from being a luxury, being fitter and stronger means we will have *more* capacity to cope, should such demands arise.

In the next chapter, I will be introducing you to the Foundational 10 Movements. This science-backed and common-sense approach has been tried and tested, both by myself in my own journey to strengthening my body, and by those who I work with. The benefits of these movements extend into every aspect of life, and will give you more capacity and energy to do other things. I found that they addressed many of my body's weaker spots that had been neglected for years – and their simplicity means I do not have to think too much about them any more, removing any anxiety about how I can remain strong and healthy. My aim is not only that your physical health will improve, but also that you will feel more relaxed and confident about the future.

Setting your strength compass

If, like me, you enjoy the great outdoors, you probably think you know your way around a map. I wonder how many of us reading these words have had moments when we've refused to accept that we're lost and continue to hope that our surroundings will miraculously start to match up to what the map says. It's all too easy to convince ourselves that we know best, or blindly hope that just over the horizon or around the next corner the directions will make sense and we will be justified in our confidence. But in strength training it's essential to have a good look at that map and understand your journey – from your starting point to your destination. Because, as you saw from the strength map in Chapter 1, getting lost in this case could mean injury, poor health and perhaps frailty. In previous chapters, we've talked about our destination point of a stronger older age many times; let's now turn our attention to the starting point on our strength journey.

At the start of any journey, you will need to be realistic in setting your direction of travel. Crucial to this is our initial choice of strength activity, which for novices, will mean easing in gently. Before getting started, I will give you tips on how to prepare your body for increased challenge via strengthening your connective tissue, learning movements and mobilising joints before progressing. I strongly encourage everyone to invest a little time reflecting on their current strength levels and their history, if any, with strength training.

> Make a note here of your experiences of exercise and strength training. It will help you later in this chapter when you are deciding what starting point best suits you.
> - When was the last time you exercised?
>   (This can include any exercise, such as running, cycling, swimming, tennis, yoga or pilates etc)
> - How often do you exercise a week?
> - When was the last time you participated in strength training?
>   (This can include training undertaken at home, at the gym, in group classes or working with a personal trainer)
> - How many times a week do you practise strength training?

This is an essential foundation to building muscle well, because all too often, an injury can occur in the initial stages of new exercise (strength training especially) if your body's structures are unaccustomed to the increased or different forces created, as discussed in Chapter 5.

Those who are new to strength training should include longer periods of lighter-intensity work to allow adaptation within all the structures that are affected by it (nervous system, bones, connective tissue and of course skeletal muscle). For example, a muscle will often respond quickly to strength training, whilst connective tissues take longer to strengthen, as their rate of adaptation is slower. Although you might feel frustrated and keen to progress to more intense training in the early phase of your strength journey, it is important to remain mindful of this fact and only train as hard as the weakest part of your whole system – i.e. your connective tissues – permits.

The good news here is that by reading the map before we set out, we are significantly decreasing any form of injury whilst increasing our strength.

Shaping your future

Body shape can refer to the type of body we have in relation to postural traits, height, broadness, length of our limbs and even our shoe size. Many of these are inherited features that we can do very little to change. If you are setting out with a goal to radically transform your body shape in middle age, you need to think again, unless it involves drastic fat loss. Whether we like it or not, we are pretty much stuck with the frame we have, albeit with the capacity to improve certain aspects. Often when working with people in midlife, I witness the light-bulb moment when they realise that even a perfect strength training programme will not bring about a drastic alteration to their general appearance.

The strength-training approach I advocate will often lead to improved muscle tone and some increased muscle mass, but it's not going to be as dramatic a change as those seen in bodybuilding.

Rowers row because they are generally tall with long limbs, providing the ability to generate the leverage that is essential to rowing. Rugby players are selected to play in the pack because they are big or broad-shouldered. Elite runners are often thin and wiry. There are always exemptions to these rules, but such activities attract certain body types – the activity itself is not responsible for developing a certain body shape. As we will be exploring, we can do lots to improve our strength, posture and ability to move well. However, we must be realistic in recognising that we are improving the cards our genes have dealt us, not drastically changing them.

Do you have a particular postural trait in your family? Are the women or men in your family generally a particular height or frame? Because, as we are about to learn, understanding such tendencies can help us tailor our strength training to suit our individual needs.

What's your type?

Dr William Sheldon first defined the three main body types in the 1940s. His work outlined the main physical characteristics of each group; the tall and lanky *ectomorph*, the rounder and softer *endomorph* – who may carry more body fat – and the more muscular *mesomorph*, who generally have slimmer hips and carry less fat. Although you may conform to one of these categories, nothing in life is ever this clearcut. In fact, we now know that we are likely to be a combination or hybrid of a couple or all three types.

When I started thinking about my own body shape at the beginning of my recovery, I found I was a mix of several types. I am predisposed to a mesomorph upper body, but, as I tend to store fat more readily in my legs, I would characterise my lower body as endomorph. Knowing my body type has focused my training on finding ways of keeping my legs strong without aggravating my back condition, which means that I never miss leg training day! I'm now conscious of the fact that, if I did, the muscles of my lower limbs would be infiltrated by fat to the detriment of my muscle. When I discuss the issue of body types with patients, they nearly always recall a family trait or relative that looked a certain 'family way'. Perhaps your family has a particular jawline, recognisable posture or walking gait, that seems to be shared between generations. Or perhaps a tendency to store fat in a certain body region? The good news is that even if there are some things that you can't change completely, diet and exercise can often help. A thin person can gain muscle. An overweight person can improve their fat-to-muscle ratio. A muscular person can improve their flexibility and cardiovascular fitness. But only if they are consistent in their approach to healthy diet and strength training, and understand their personal body type.

Fast responder

Do you know people who just seem to be naturally good at exercise without trying? Worse still, do they look lean or muscular and actually do very little exercise compared to you? Perhaps in school there was a person who was intuitively best in a certain sport and had an incredible build in their teens. You may be pleased to hear that it is far more important to finish strong in life than to have your athletic high-water mark at school. Frankly, even if you were, as I sometimes was, the last to be chosen for a school sports team, you will always win if you finish strong. My moment of realisation came shortly after my 18th birthday, when I joined the fire service training school. The act of moving to London and training with individuals who were generally 10 years older, with completely different life experiences, was the best education I could have had and reset some of the negative self-perceptions I was still holding onto from my school days.

Your athletic high-water mark may be yet to come. I know mine was.

The take-home here is that although we can't change our frames, what we hang on those frames is absolutely up for grabs. Everyone is born with certain predispositions to distribution patterns for not only fat, but also for different muscle fibre types, which again affects our innate ability to be strong. Someone with a greater amount of fast-twitch fibres than slow-twitch fibres is more likely to be better at strength and power-type exercise, whereas someone with more slow-twitch fibres will be better at endurance-type activities. As we know from Chapter 3, it is important for endurance-focused individuals to also build their fast-twitch fibres. And for those who have historically focused on strength-training activities, to include cardiovascular exercise. The same principles are true for all of us in middle age, in that we need to become more *hybrid* in our approach to physical training.

Hybrid workout

During my recruit firefighter training, there was a heavy emphasis on hybrid fitness exercise sessions, which included circuits with names like the 'dirty dozen' or 'filthy fifteen'. These combined aerobic-type activities with resistance training, which targeted all regions of the body and were effective in preparing us for the physical rigours of firefighting. These classes were great at getting younger people fitter quickly, and addressing potential weaker areas of body movement.

Whatever our natural body type, such information is gold dust as it enables us to develop an approach that works not just on our strength but also addresses our potential weaknesses. What this approach exemplifies is the value of working not just on the things we find comforting, familiar or easy; identifying and targeting the chinks in our armour will also be a great advantage in the long run. Arguably the greatest boxer of all time, Muhammad Ali, would relish the opportunity to work on his weaknesses in training camps. We now know that with hindsight he continued in boxing for far too long, with tragic consequences for his long-term health.[1] However, his training philosophy still stands up. Famously, he would spend months looking terrible in training, deliberately working on what he felt were his weaknesses when compared to his next opponent in the ring, so much so that his coaches and family would be in constant fear of him losing or getting hurt. However, Ali was certain that resisting the temptation to look good whilst working on his weakness would in fact give him an advantage. It was this philosophy of chosing the path of most resistance, in my opinion, that made him one of the greats.

I am sure we can all relate to the mindset of sticking to the things we find undemanding and familiar, including our exercise choices. The problem with this is that we will only be strong in a few movements and weak in others. To be strong in life, we need to be work on all major body movements, not just the ones we are already good at.

What do you think your body type is? Is it one or a mixture of the three listed above? Do you tend to stick to particular exercises or are you really strong in a particular movement and not in others? Are you good at running, cycling, swimming, or yoga, and tend to stick to that?

By being honest with ourselves about such matters, we will be able to build an age-resistant suit that will truly have us covered. There is no point working on our upper bodies, whilst ignoring our lower body, or vice versa. This would be like a firefighter pairing a fire-resistant jacket with plastic leggings (happily the fire service issued us with matching fire-resistant leggings in the early 90s!).

In the next section, you will have the opportunity to reflect on where you currently sit on your strength journey. You may feel frustrated to be easing in slowly, but remember that we have the luxury of time with us, because our goals are not set for next month or next year but for the next 30 years.

Before you make a start

For the vast majority of us at any age, increasing our levels of exercise – including strength training – will be beneficial for our health and wellbeing. There are, however, a few situations in which an individual should seek their doctor's advice prior to increasing their exercise levels or trying a new activity. Below is a questionnaire often used in the fitness and health industries to determine an individual's readiness to exercise.

Before starting a new activity – including any of the exercises contained within this book – you should first ask yourself these questions:

- Has your doctor ever said that you have a heart condition and that you should only do physical activity recommended by a doctor?
- Do you feel pain in your chest when you do physical activity?
- In the past month, have you had chest pain when you were not doing physical activity?
- Do you lose your balance because of dizziness, or do you ever lose consciousness?
- Do you have a bone or joint problem that could be made

worse by a change in your physical activity?

- Is your doctor currently prescribing drugs for your blood pressure or heart condition?
- Do you know of any other reason why you should not do physical activity?

If you answer 'yes' to any of the questions above, you should consult your doctor for advice on starting any new strength activity. In many cases, with some guidance from your doctor, you will still be able to exercise.

If your doctor agrees that you are able to start strength training but have pre-existing injuries or a joint condition that might stop you from doing some of the Foundational 10 Movements, you should consult with a qualified fitness professional or a physical practitioner such as an osteopath or a physiotherapist. They will be able to offer alternative ways of strengthening any movements to better suit your individual capability.

If you've had surgery or are returning from an injury or illness that has kept you inactive or are in any doubt about your readiness to start exercise, please consult your doctor.

If you have had a C-section or have had a child and have not conducted core and pelvic floor rehab, then you should consider doing some pelvic floor/core rehabilitation with a qualified Pilates teacher prior to starting these prep stages.

If you are pregnant or could be pregnant, you should seek your doctor's advice on starting any new exercise or activity such as strength training.

Identifying your start point

How to prepare for the Foundational 10 Movements

You'll be pleased to hear that building strength does not have to be stressful. It is in our long-term health interest to take any emotional worry or stress out of what our exercise choices should be. The beauty of these 10 movements is that they remove any uncertainty – you can relax in the knowledge that you have it covered. All you need to do is turn up!

The main factors that decide your starting point are the amount of experience you have had in strength training and your general physical condition and activity levels.

The section below outlines the three levels of strength I use to help people find their starting point. Look at the descriptions for each and see which one you recognise or resonate with. With each, I recommend how much time to spend at this stage.

Level 1

Familiarisation and readying your system

1 month

This is for you if you:
- have no experience with strength training;
- are coming back from a long spell of inactivity;
- have not exercised with regularity for more than six months but are occasionally active; and
- you are free from injury and in good health.

You may well find your muscles have detrained to a point that any exercise seems daunting. Therefore, we need to reframe your expectations. It's a question of first strengthening the entire body before focusing on your muscles. This means you need to increase your exercise levels more generally to help accustom your body to being more physically active. This will gently strengthen your body first and provide a better starting point for strength training.

You will be greatly served by spending one month using the Minimal Loading Programme on page 126. You also need to engage in more general exercise, such as brisk walking, swimming, gardening or cycling, which will help get your body moving again. This will be sufficient to increase your overall strength, enabling you to progress to the Foundational 10 Movements, which are described in Chapter 7.

Note: The static (otherwise known as isometric) elements of the exercises will ensure your muscles AND connective tissues have enough time to strengthen before progressing.

If after one month (+ or – one to two weeks) all has gone well and you are free from injury and overt fatigue, you are ready to progress to the Foundational 10 Movements.

Level 2

Familiarisation and readying your system

2 weeks

This starting point is for you if:

- you have done little or no strength training in the last six months;
- you are free from injury and in good health; and
- you are exercising or active regularly.

Even if you have done a little strength training in the past, you still need to go back to basics. However, you are likely to regain some of your previous strength more quickly than a complete beginner. You should spend two weeks (+ or – one week, depending on how you are responding) using the Minimal Loading Programme overleaf. This will remind your nervous system of the movement patterns you have previously experienced, or indeed teach it some new ones. It will also get your joints accustomed to the planes of movement and full range of motion that will be required when you start to strength-train. You should continue with the other exercise activities you are already doing.

Note: If you complete this period and are free from injury, pain and fatigue, it is time to progress to the Foundational 10 Movements.

Level 3
Familiarisation
2 weeks

You are at this level if you:

- have consistently engaged in circuit training with weights or gym machines for years and continue to do so;
- have consistently engaged in bodybuilding or strength work either at home or in a gym and continue to do so; and
- you are free from injury and in good health.

In your case, it won't take much time to prepare your body. You will benefit from two weeks of incorporating the stretching and mobilisation elements of my Minimal Loading Programme below into your normal routine. You will also find the 'going through the gears' approach helpful to adopt in your training (see FAQs in Chapter 7). Take a look at the Foundational 10 Movements to see if there's anything there that you are not familiar with. If you don't recognise something, perhaps try a few weeks of minimal loading within the movements that you might not have done before. Consider incorporating the movements into your existing cardiovascular training schedule and see how you feel. You should focus more on deciding what your training week will look like and perhaps try some different approaches that will best suit your lifestyle.

Note: For you, it's not so much that you are experiencing new things; it's more about shifting your focus from the short to longer term.

Starting out: Minimal Loading Programme

Aim to do all the elements below once a week. You can split the exercises across several days or do them in one session.

- Always warm up before you start. This can be a brisk 5-minute walk around the block whilst breathing deeply and swinging your arms.

- Ensure you leave at least 2 minutes between bouts of effort.
- Always warm down, relax and stretch when you finish.

Scan the QR code above for a demonstration of my suggested stretches.

Upper body

Horizontal shoulder push: Focus on the muscles in your chest and muscle on rear of your upper arms.

Wall press: Whilst standing, hold out your arms in front of you and place them on a wall. Your weight should now be held between your feet and your hands – similar to a plank position. However, you should allow a slight bend at the elbows, feeling your body weight through your hands.

Whilst holding this static press-up position, count to 30 and then take a break for 2 minutes. Do this 3 times. If this seems easy, you can try the same move, but with more of a bend at the elbows, which will make it more challenging.

Level up: If this version begins to feel too easy, progress to a static box press-up position. To do this, position yourself on all fours, with your arms straight and your body weight resting on bent knees. Keep your back flat so that your body is in a straight line, with your bottom tucked in. Continue with the same 3 sets of 30-second counts, with a 2-minute rest between.

If the box press-up becomes easy, progress to holding a standard press-up position statically with a slight bend at the elbows.

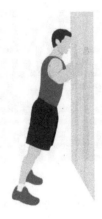

Wall press

Horizontal shoulder pull: Focus on the muscles in your upper back and the front of your arms.

Static towel door hold: First, stand with your arms held straight out in front of you and your feet shoulder width apart.

Sling a towel around an immovable object, grip with both hands and then lean back. (I like to place a towel around a banister – but you could also use a door handle, or close a knotted towel into a doorframe using the unknotted end to grip). When using any household furniture or fittings, ensure you test they are safe to use first.

Standing with feet shoulder width apart, grip the towel with both hands and lean back, keeping a slight bend at your knees and a straight back and looking straight forward.

Keep your arms straight and hold for the count of 30, then break for 2 minutes. Repeat this 3 times.

Level up: You can add time in 10-second increments per week. When this feels easy, you can progress by doing the same movement with a slight bend at your elbows.

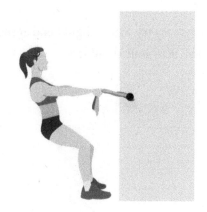

Static towel door hold

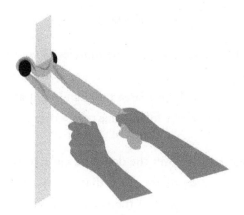

How to secure your towel

Vertical shoulder push: Focus on your shoulders and posterior arm muscles.

Wall hold: Standing facing a wall, place your hands on it and walk them down until your chest is parallel to the ground – you will be looking at the floor.

Walk your feet back until your hips and back are in a straight line and 90 degrees to the wall. Allow your body weight to lean into the wall with your upper body weight going through your hands, arms and shoulders. Hold this position whilst counting to 30 and then rest for 2 minutes. Repeat this 3 times.

Level up: If this seems easy try with a slight bend at the elbow or adjust your feet until you feel it in your shoulders.

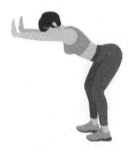

Wall hold

Vertical shoulder pull: Focus on the muscles of your upper back and below your shoulders.

Vertical shoulder pull: Take a large towel and tie it at one end using a simple granny knot, made by folding one corner over the over and pulling it tight.

Place the knotted end over the door and close it. Let the other end hang down on the side of the door that opens away from you, not towards you, i.e. when you pull the towel it should further close the door. Pull up a chair to sit on, facing the door.

Sitting up straight, reach above your head with both arms straight and firmly grab the two corners of the towel – your hands should be about shoulder width apart. Make sure that any slack has been taken up and the towel is tight.

Then, with straight arms, pull downwards with your shoulders until you feel your weight in the chair lighten slightly. Hold this position, keeping your arms straight and head forward. You will feel your weight in your hands, upper back and or course glutes.

Hold for 3 lots of 30 seconds.

Level up: Add 10-second increments to this exercise per week. When it feels too easy, holding the position with a slight bend at the elbows.

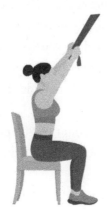

Vertical shoulder pull

Core and lower back

Wall or chair plank: Use a wall or stable chair to hold your body in a ridged plank-like position with your body weight between your forearms and toes. You should start with the wall plank and progress to the chair plank if it becomes easy.

Always check the stability of any furniture if using it for this purpose.

Hold for 3 sets of 20 seconds, adding 5–10 seconds per session.

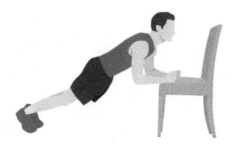

Chair plank

Lower body

Wall sits: Place your back flat against a wall and slowly allow your bum to slide towards the floor until your thighs are just above right angles – imagine there is a chair below you (you can place a stool or chair under you if this makes you feel more confident). Essentially, you are simply going to allow your back to slide down the wall to sit in the imaginary or real chair.

Hold this position for the count of 30 and then stand up from the wall and rest for 2 minutes. Repeat this 3 times.

Level up: When this feels easy, add 5–10 seconds per session.

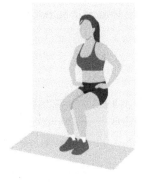

Wall sit

Hips

Hip thrusts: Lie on the floor with your back flat, knees bent and feet shoulderwidth apart. Bring your pelvis up in a thrusting movement so that it is in line with your thighs, with your weight carried between your shoulders and feet. Hold the uppermost position while your hips are up.

Aim to hold this position for 3 sets of 10–20 seconds, adding 5–10 seconds per session.

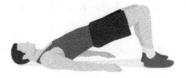

Hip thrust

Grip

Towel twist: Roll a hand towel until it matches your hand size. With your arms straight and outstretched, grasp it firmly with both hands, then alternate rotating one wrist downwards and the other upwards to create a kind of wringing movement.

Start with 3 sets of 10 seconds, adding 2 seconds each time.

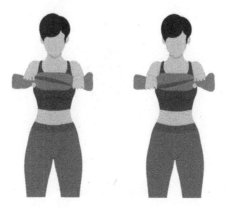

Towel twist

Farmer's hold: Fill two shopping bags, suitcases or rucksacks with some food cans and practise holding them whilst standing. You can also use weights or kettle bells, if you have them.

Your arms should be straight and your shoulders in parallel with your ears. Keep your back straight at all times, including when picking up the bags.

If after 30 seconds you are not feeling any resistance through your forearms or hands, try adding more cans to your bag. You should feel the weight in your hands and the rest of your body, including your feet.

Hold for 3 lots of 30 seconds, and add 10 second increments per week.

Level up: When this feels too easy, consider adding some extra weight to the bags or use heavier weights if you have them.

Note: Some people like to do this movement with their back to the wall to keep it nice and straight. If using a chair for this exercise, ensure that your back is straight and supported by the chair back.

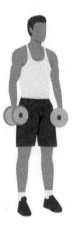

Farmer's hold

Stretches

Stretch the area you trained, without fail, at the end of *every* session.

Once stretched, consider taking 5 minutes to rest. Sit or lie in a position of comfort, close your eyes and concentrate on breathing in deeply through the nose and out through the mouth, exhaling slowly. Some people find it helpful to count steadily from 1 to 5 when breathing in and out.

For a demonstration of stretches covering the upper and lower body, core, hips and grip, go to:

Equipment list

The items below are optional and is by no means essential.

- Exercise bands/ grip resistance bands
- Adjustable weight sets (I recommend a pair of adjustable dumb-bells if starting out)
- Pull-up bar (various models including doorframe, free-standing or wall mounted are available)
- Alternative option: suspension systems (door, wall or ceiling mounted and consisting of long straps with handles that can be secured to doorframes or other anchor points)
- Door or ceiling anchor points are another sensible purchase if starting out (for using with suspension systems, exercise bands or towels).

Note on equipment: When starting out, you can strength-train without the need for any equipment. However, as you progress, I would suggest you invest in some of the equipment above. I personally feel that exercise bands, anchor points or pull-up bars are a great investment for getting stronger at home. That said, you only need to invest in new equipment as and when you get stronger, once you surpass what you can achieve with your body weight and the use of towels!

7

The Foundational 10 Movements

'I am glad I am not strong any more.'
No one, ever

Ernest Hemingway apparently once said that we all die twice. Once when we are buried and again when our names are spoken for the last time. I believe it's possible to die before these two events, when in old age we lose our physical ability to live independently or without care. Whilst there are circumstances that might lead to this situation that are beyond our control, the majority of us can avoid or significantly delay this death of independence by preserving our strength and the quality of our muscles.

Far from being a privilege of the rich and healthy, athleticism and vitality in older age are attainable for everyone. We simply need to commit to our own strength journey and realise our goals with consistency, effort, and smart training.

Having got this far in understanding the science of strength training and finding your individual starting point, you are well on your way to a stronger future. I encourage you to view the information in this chapter as the foundation for living your best life deep into old age. Think of the initial 12-week phase of this plan as a kind of 'Couch to 5k' for strength. I call this the Foundation and Familiarisation Phase, in that, during this time, you will have improved your strength, increased your joint mobility, identified strength imbalances and created a place and time in your life for strength training.

Using the Foundational 10 Movements, you will see how easy it is to track your strength whilst incorporating training into your week. If you are not ready to start the 12-week Foundation and Familiarisation Phase, that's fine too. I encourage you to find a way of starting training that suits you, either by using the Minimal Loading Programme (page 126) or perhaps by committing to as little as a few minutes a day of strength snacking – more on this later. Minutes will accumulate into hours, which can get you stronger over time, whilst also preparing your body for when you are ready to do more. The most important thing is to make a start.

One of the main pillars of strength training is working towards a specific goal. We need to establish what we are hoping to gain with strength training (think back to the reasons you noted down on your strength bucket list in Chapter 1). My own list includes being able to climb Ben Nevis or any other mountain I choose, run around the garden with my grandchildren or simply continue to take part in the sports or pastimes that I enjoy as I age.

The Foundational 10 Movements were developed with the following criteria in mind:

- Stability: to build body-wide, functional muscle, strength and power
- Safety: to avoid fatigue and injury
- Simplicity: to democratise strength training and make it accessible for anyone
- Sustainability: to allow busy people to embed strength training in their lives.

Before we explore the exercise themselves, there are a few key things that you should know first.

The three types of muscle contraction

There are three main types of muscle contraction: *concentric*, *eccentric* and *isometric*. Each type has a set of unique characteristics and offers singular advantages in terms of developing or maintaining strength.

Ideally, we want to become stronger in all contraction types. *All* three types should be incorporated into a longer-term strength-training plan, because being strong in all types of contraction will protect us from injury in old age.

1. Concentric contraction: shortening strength

A concentric contraction occurs when we shorten a muscle.

The bicep curl is a good example of this (when we shorten the muscles on the front of our arms by bringing our hands towards our shoulders). When doing this with nothing in our hands, this is usually easy, with only gravity and the weight of our arms to overcome in order to achieve the movement. If we were to do this with something in our hands (such as an exercise band or a dumb-bell) the same movement would require more force and effort to overcome the weight of the object in bringing the hand towards the shoulder.

2. Eccentric contraction: lengthening strength

An eccentric contraction occurs when we lengthen a muscle under load.

If we bring our hands up to our shoulders, then let them fall to our sides with no effort to slow them down, there will be an eccentric lengthening of the muscle on the front of our arms. If we deliberately slow the speed of our hands returning to our sides whilst holding a weight, this becomes an eccentric *contraction* i.e. a lengthening of the muscle *under a load*. Interestingly, this lengthening under tension places a higher load on the muscles than the other contraction types.

We can harness the benefits of this contraction by deliberately slowing this phase down. This is called a 'negative rep', because we place as much or more emphasis on the *lowering* element of the exercise. This would mean a slower emphasis on the lowering phase of a squat, lunge or pull-up – or a slower lowering of your chest to the floor in a press-up. You may also recall from Chapter 5 (see: '*Strengthening our braking system will protect us*' on page 96) that there is a great deal of older-age benefit to be gained from including negative reps in our strength training in terms of strength preservation and injury prevention.

3. Isometric contraction: static strength

An isometric contraction involves the contraction of a muscle without shortening or lengthening.

This type of contraction is incredibly useful in helping you keep a muscle strong if you have injured a joint and you are unable to engage it in concentric or eccentric contractions, which are more dymanic. It is also invaluable in strengthening our connective tissues in the initial phases of strength training or after returning from a long period of inactivity as it does not overload the body. Examples of how we can use this contraction type include wall-sits and the static farmer's hold. In fact, any movement, such as a press-up or squat at the mid-point, can be held statically.

Periodisation

Periodisation in strength-training programmes refers to how we manipulate different variables to maximise strength and minimise injury or fatigue – this means adjusting things like rest periods; how often we do an exercise; how hard we make it; and what type of exercise we do. Strength and conditioning coaches often use timed programmes that help an athlete peak at major competitions. Our goal, however, is not to peak but to have consistency of strength throughout our lives.

I draw on my own strength story in this book because in preparing for the ageing game, we need to be ready to respond to yet unknown challenges that, in many ways, mirror those faced by a firefighter. They too need the ability to be consistently fit, strong and ready to respond. They do not train to peak periodically for a sporting competition, because their competition – in the form of an emergency incident – can happen at any time. They have to train to be fit and strong *enough* year round. Similarly, when training for older-age strength, we need to keep turning up consistently because in doing so, we will be ready for any challenges with *enough* reserves of energy and strength to call on.

Reps, sets and rest periods

Repetitions or 'reps', are the number of times we repeat a given exercise. Therefore, if you repeat an exercise 10 times, you would be completing '10 reps'.

Sets refer to how many groups of reps we need to complete. For example, completing 4 lots of 10 reps would be expressed as '4 sets of 10 repetitions of an exercise'

Rest periods are as important to get right as actual strength training. This is because our bodies need to recover fully after we have worked it. It means we get the most benefit from working our muscles and nervous system when they are recharged and ready to go (remember the underlying rules about avoiding burnout and fatigue explored in Chapter 5). I recommend at least 2 minutes rest between sets. If you are tempted to cut this period short, don't be – it would be like only half charging your e-bike or electric car: you are going to break down halfway through your journey and not enjoy the feeling of power.

Note: The number of reps we perform can be manipulated to help us build functional muscle, strength or power - more on this later.

Choosing your starting point and how hard it should feel

You will see that there is a spectrum of versions with varying difficulties within the Foundational 10 Movements, from which you will choose your starting point for each. If starting out on the Foundation and Familiarisation Phase, you can find which variation of a movement will be your starting point by first trying to perform 10 reps. If you are struggling to complete all 10, then select the next movement variation down – you can also adopt one of the corresponding Minimal Loading Programme movements in Chapter 6 as your starting point for any of the movements. If you can do 10 reps easily, you should try a more challenging version of the movement as your starting point. If using weights, adjust accordingly until you can complete 10 reps.

It should feel moderately hard by the time you complete the tenth rep (on a difficulty scale, it should feel like a 6–7 out of 10), meaning you should feel as though you could do another 3 reps. Or put another way, 3 reps away from being unable to perform another rep and having to stop. Your goal should be to perform all 10 reps smoothly in each set.

The Movements

I encourage you to view the Foundational 10 Movements as a kind of shorthand to strength. Knowing how busy life gets, I have only included the movements that are truly worthy of our effort and time.

In midlife, our lives can look very different week to week, which might mean that you can't complete the entire programme as often as you had planned. A pivotal life moment came for me when I gave myself permission to be middle-aged and train towards realistic strength goals. If I am pushed for time one week and don't complete the training I had planned, I'm relaxed about it. We are going to have good days or weeks when we are bossing it, and other periods when we are barely able to cope with work/family responsibility, let alone exercise. Even a few minutes spent strengthening these movements will still be building towards strength in older age. Missing a session or a movement *is not a failure*, if over the long term you are to be consistent.

I will explain each movement in detail, including how to do them and what the key benefits will be once you've incorporated them into your life.

Upper body

1. Horizontal shoulder push
2. Horizontal shoulder pull
3. Vertical shoulder push
4. Vertical shoulder pull

Core and lower back

5. Plank

Lower body

6. Squat
7. Hip thrust
8. Lunge

Grip

9. Grip and lean, or grip and hang
10. Farmer's hold or walk

1. Horizontal shoulder push

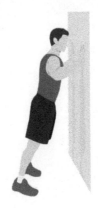

Wall press

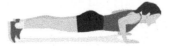

Box or standard press-up

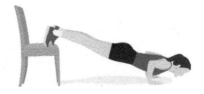

Elevated feet press-up

What?

The horizontal shoulder push targets the muscles in the chest, the rear of upper arm and the front shoulder in the horizonal plane of movement (if you want to get technical, the specific muscles this movement targets are the pectorals, triceps and front deltoids). Think: a 'pushing away' movement with your hands to the front of your body.

Why?
- Good for shoulder stability
- Improves your ability to safely push up or get off the floor unaided
- Prevents falling by improving your ability to quickly reach out and grab onto something
- Great for sports and recreational activities into older age
- Builds self-defence, self-confidence and self-reliance.

How?
Choose your starting point:
- Wall press
- Box or standard press-up
- Elevated feet press-up (optional use of rucksack).

Wall press: Stand facing the wall. Put your arms out in front of you and place your palms on the wall, keeping a slight bend in your elbows. You should be holding your body weight between your hands and feet. Bend your elbows until your chest is 2 inches from the wall, keeping your back straight and stomach muscles tight. Then push away, straightening your arms to the starting position.

Box press: Position yourself on the floor in a tabletop-like posture, with your hands below your shoulders and knees below your hips. Keep your hands at the 12 o'clock position, distributing your weight evenly between your hands and knees. Allow your elbows to bend until your chest is 2 inches off the floor, keeping your back straight and stomach muscles tight. Then push upwards to the starting position.

Press-up: Place your hands on the floor, slightly more than shoulderwidth apart. Create a straight line from your head to your heels, with your toes touching the ground so that you are holding your weight through your hands and feet. Keep your arms straight and try not to allow your body to sag. Bend your elbows until your chest is 2 inches off the floor, keeping your back straight and stomach muscles tight. Then push upwards to the starting position.

Elevated feet press-up: On all fours, raise your feet behind you onto a sofa or chair, forming a press-up position with the only difference being the slant of your body. Hold your weight between your hands and feet, keeping your back straight and your body at this slightly declined angle. Bend your elbows until your chest is 2 inches off the floor. Keep your stomach muscles tight. Push upwards to the starting position.

Note: If the elevated feet press-up version is likely to aggravate your lower back, consider wearing a weighted rucksack to add more difficulty to the standard press-up instead.

You can progress from these versions of the press-up to using free weights and a bench, or a bench-press machine, in a gym, with the advice of a qualified fitness professional.

Super set: Pair this with Movement 2 – horizontal shoulder pull overleaf.

2. Horizontal shoulder pull

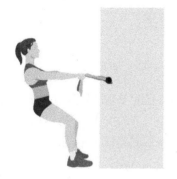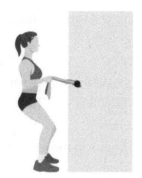

Horizontal towel pull

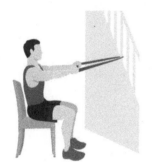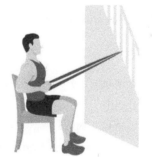

Exercise band pull

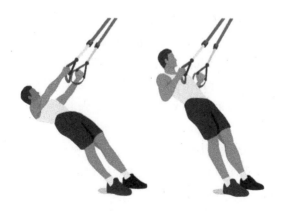

Suspension system

What?

This movement targets the muscles in the back, the rear shoulders, and the front of the arms (the latimus dorsi, deltoids and biceps). Think: outstretched arms, pulling towards your chest.

Why?

- Good for shoulder stability
- Improves your ability to pull yourself up from the floor or climb stairs
- Improves the posture of your upper back and neck and protects them from the strain induced by prolonged sitting
- Limits injury from falling
- Great for sports and recreational activities into older age
- Improves your ability to pick things up from the floor
- Maintains your ability to pick up and carry your shopping.

How?

Choose your starting point:

- Towel pull
- Exercise band pull
- Suspension system (requires equipment).

Towel pull: Loop a small towel across and under the handles of an open door (see diagram opposite). Grip the towel with both hands and straighten your arms, keeping your back straight. Lower your bum by bending your knees by a few inches, with your feet below/in line with them. Keeping your feet still, pull your hands towards you, your elbows coming to your sides and your body moving gently towards the towel. Allow your arms to straighten as your body gently moves away from the towel back to the starting position. To progress, simply increase the bend in your knees and place your feet closer to the door.

Exercise band pull: You can do this standing or seated. Wrap the band around a banister at chest height. Grip each side of the band and pull your hands towards your chest, bending your elbows to your sides, keeping your torso straight and as stationary as possible. Allow your arms to straighten as your hands return to your starting point. Progress this movement by opting for a thicker band.

Suspension system: This requires a home or gym exercise suspension system that consists of handles and straps. If using at home, secure your system to the top of a doorframe or other anchor points so that the handles and straps hang down (see Chapter 6: *Equipment list – suspension systems and anchor points*). Standing up straight, grip each handle, making sure that there is no slack in the straps. Then lean your body back slightly with straight arms. Keeping your feet still, pull your hands towards your chest, bending your elbows to your sides and keeping your body straight. Allow your arms to straighten and your hands return to your starting point. To progress, allow the angle of your lean to increase whilst keeping your feet planted and your body straight.

You can progress from these versions of the movement by using a seated rowing machine in a gym, with the advice of a qualified fitness professional.

Super set: Pair this move with Movement 1 – horizontal shoulder push (page 144).

How to secure your towel

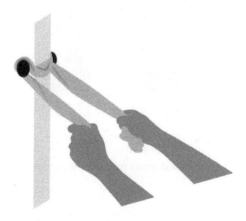

3. Vertical shoulder push

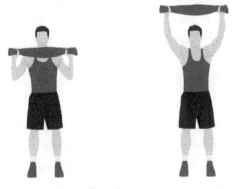

Towel press

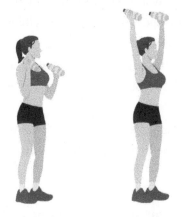

Household object (e.g. water bottle) press

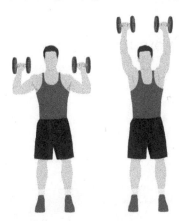

Weighted press (requires weights)

What?

This movement targets the muscles in the shoulders and the rear of the arms or 'bingo wings' (the deltoids and triceps). Think: reaching above your head to place an object on a high shelf.

Why?

- Good for shoulder stability
- Good for lifting upwards, for example, placing things on shelves or in an overhead cupboard
- Protects your neck and shoulder posture
- Prevents shoulder injuries
- Improves your ability to decorate or clean your home in older age
- Builds self-defence, self-confidence and self-reliance.

How?

Choose your starting point:

- Towel press
- Household object press (requires water bottle)
- Weighted press (requires equipment).

Towel press: You can either do this seated in a stable chair or standing with your feet shoulderwidth apart. Roll or fold a large towel tightly so that you can grip it firmly with both hands, shoulder-width apart. Start with your towel at chest height, your palms facing forwards and your elbows bent to your side. Push the towel upwards and straight above your head using your shoulders. Straighten your arms but do not fully lock out your elbows. Keeping the tension between your hands whilst gripping the towel, bend your elbows to lower the towel to chest height. Your hands should be at shoulder level.

Household object press: Carefully select household objects that offer some weight and good grip. You can either do this seated on a stable chair or standing with your feet shoulderwidth apart. I recommend using water bottles in the first instance. Start with your water bottles at shoulder height, your palms facing forwards and in line with your ears. Push upwards and straight above your head using your shoulders. Straighten your arms but do not fully lock out your elbows. Bend your elbows to lower the bottles to shoulder level.

Weighted press: You can either do this seated on a stable chair or standing with your feet shoulderwidth apart. I suggest you use a set of adjustable dumb-bells for this version of the movement (see Chapter 6: *Equipment list*). Start with your dumb-bells at shoulder height, palms facing forwards and in line with your ears. Push upwards and straight above your head using your shoulders. Straighten your arms but do not fully lock out your elbows. Bending your elbows, lower your hands, allowing the bottles to return to shoulder level.

You can progress from these versions of the movement by using a shoulder press machine in a gym, with the advice of a qualified fitness professional.

Super set: Pair this with Movement 4 – vertical shoulder pull (instructions overleaf).

4. Vertical shoulder pull

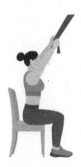

Towel pull-up

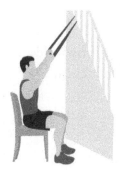 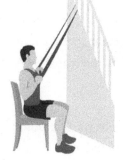

Exercise band pull-down

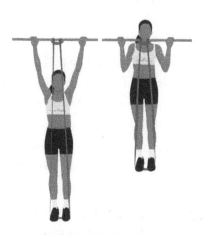

Band-assisted pull-up

What?

This movement targets the muscles in the back and the front of the arms, as well as the larger muscles of the shoulder joints (between the shoulder blades and the smaller spinal muscles of the upper back), in the vertical plane of movement (the latimus dorsi). Think: pulling yourself up and over a high wall.

Why?

- Good for shoulder stability
- Improves your ability to climb stairs or pull yourself up from the floor
- Protects your long-term upper-back and neck posture
- Limits injury from falling
- Great for sports and recreational activities into older age
- Works the whole body and builds grip strength.

How?

Choose your starting point:

- Towel pull-up
- Exercise band pull-down
- Band-assisted pull-up (requires pull-up bar and exercise bands)

Towel pull-up: Tie a granny knot at the end of a large towel by folding one corner over the other, making sure to pull it tight. Place the knotted end over the door and close it. Let the unknotted end of the towel hang down on the side of the door that opens away from you, not towards you, i.e. pulling the towel should further close the door. Pull the towel downwards to take up any slack. Sitting up straight in a chair, with your knees at right angles and your feet directly below them reach above your head with both arms and firmly grab the two corners of the towel – your hands should be shoulderwidth apart. Now pull your hands downwards – bending your elbows until your hands are at shoulder level. You will naturally stand up. Try to use your upper body to pull as much as possible in this movement until you have stood up. Still gripping the towel with both hands, bend your knees to lower your bum towards the chair whilst allowing your elbows to straighten. Control the lowering phase of this movement back to the seated position as much as you can with your upper body. Do not slump back into the chair.

To progress, place your feet further away from you, which will focus more of the effort required to stand in your back and arm muscles.

Exercise band pull-down: If using an exercise band, start in the same seated position. Secure your exercise band to a high anchor-point above your head (I like to use a stair banister or a door anchor point (see Chapter 6: *Equipment list*). Then reach up with your arms straight and grasp the band with both hands. Remaining seated, bend your elbows to pull the band down until your hands are at shoulder height. Allow your elbows to straighten and your hands to return to your starting point above your head. To progress, use a thicker band.

Band-assisted pull-up: For this exercise, you will need access to a pull-up bar and exercise bands. First, loop an exercise band around the bar, letting it hang down. See instructions overleaf: *tying your band*. Pull the hanging loop of exercise band downwards and place one of your knees or feet into the loop, allowing your body weight to stretch the band downwards, then place both feet on the band. Grip the pull-up bar with your palms facing away from you. You should be under the bar with straight legs if possible, otherwise keep your knees bent. Bending your elbows, pull your chest up towards the bar and try to get your chin above it, if space allows. You will feel the boost that the exercise band offers. Try to keep your mid-section and legs still in this movement. Control the lowering of your body down to the starting position by straightening your arms. To progress, gradually reduce the thickness of the bands until you do not need them any more!

You can progress from these versions of the movement by using a lateral pull-down machine in a gym, with the advice of a qualified fitness professional.

Super set: Pair with Movement 3 – vertical shoulder push (page 144).

Tying your band

Loop the band around the bar and pull it through itself. Be sure to use the correct size.

Try different thicknesses of bands to find the one that allows you to perform the required number of reps.

5. Plank

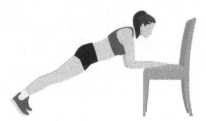

Wall or chair plank

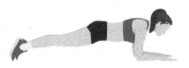

Standard plank

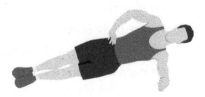

Side plank

What?

This movement targets the muscles of the midsection, including your abdominal, back and hip regions. It also has a great all-over strengthening effect.

Why?

- Strengthens the whole body
- Good for your lower-back and spinal posture
- Improves your ability to get up from a chair or the floor
- Improves your walking gait
- Protects against lower-back pain or injury
- Great for all sports and recreational activities into older age
- Protects your ability to lift and carry in older age.

How?

Choose your starting point:
- Wall or chair plank
- Standard plank
- Side plank or other variations.

Wall or chair plank: For the wall plank, stand up straight, bend your elbows and place your forearms against the wall. Your elbows should be at shoulder height with your forearms pointing vertically up the wall. Step back with both feet so that they are about shoulderwidth away from the wall. You should now be holding your weight between your toes and forearms and feeling it in your core! Keep your body straight and breathe normally. To progress, move your feet further away from the wall or try another version of this movement. For the chair plank, select a stable chair, bend your elbows and place both forearms on the flat surface of the chair, straightening both legs behind you. Your weight should be held between your toes and forearms, and your body held straight, i.e. don't allow your bum to sag downwards. Remember to breathe normally.

Standard plank: Lie face-down on a safe floor area, with your elbows directly below your shoulders and your forearms flat on the ground in front of you. Lift yourself up onto your elbows, keeping your palms flat on the floor (you should be looking down at your hands). Make a straight line from your shoulders to your heels, holding your weight between your forearms and your toes. Do not allow your bum to sag, keep your body straight and core tight and breathe normally.

Side plank: For the side plank version, lie on one side with your legs straight and one foot on top of the other. With your elbow directly below your shoulder, lift your hip up from the floor so you are supporting your weight through your elbow and the side of the foot nearest the floor.

Other plank versions: To progress you can try other versions of the standard plank such as: starting in the plank position, bend one knee and bring it towards your elbow on that side whilst supporting your weight through your forearms and the toes of the other foot. Taking care to keep your body straight and avoiding any sagging, bring your knee back to its starting position, with both feet side by side. Change sides and repeat.

For all plank versions, start with 2 sets of 30 seconds, building to 2 sets of 2 minutes before progressing to more challenging versions.

Alternative – transverse abdominal crunch: If you have back issues that make a plank difficult, you could try the transverse abdominal crunch.

Lie on the floor with your knees bent and feet flat on the ground. Place your fingertips just in front of your ears with your elbows facing forwards. Contract your core and bring your right elbow as near to your left knee as possible and back to the starting position. Repeat with your left elbow and right knee. Ensure that it's your midsection that is twisting and not your neck – always keep your head up with your chin in line with your chest. If this is too challenging, you can try moving your knee to meet your opposite elbow.

Try 3 sets of 10 each side and increase to 3 sets of 20 each side. When this becomes manageable, try increasing to 5 sets of 20 each side.

6. Squat

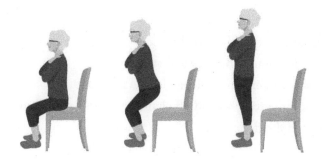

Chair squat

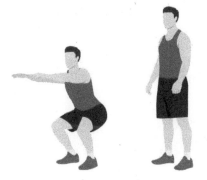

Body weight squat

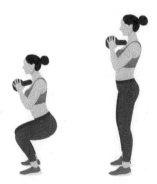

Weighted squat

What? Squatting targets all lower-limb muscles but primarily those at the front of the thighs (quadriceps), the rear of the thigh (hamstrings) and the bum (gluteal). Think: standing up from or sitting down on a chair.

Why?

- Strengthens the whole body
- Great for general balance and stability
- Good for remaining independent in older age
- Great for getting on and off chairs or toilets unaided, and getting up from the floor
- Improves your ability to climb stairs in older age
- Great for all sports and recreational activities into older age
- Improves your ability to lift and carry
- Protects against hip and knee pain or injury.

How?

Choose your starting point:

- Chair squat
- Body weight squat
- Weighted squat.

Chair squat: Select a stable chair and sit with your knees at right angles, legs shoulderwidth apart and feet directly below your knees. Then contract your thigh and bum muscles, driving upwards to the standing position with straight legs and feet facing forward. You should also be looking straight ahead. Keeping your back straight, bend your knees and allow your bum to lower towards the chair until you are back in the sitting position. Remain there for 2 seconds before repeating the movement.

Body weight squat: Start by standing with your feet shoulderwidth apart and your toes and eyes facing forwards. Bending your knees, lower your bum towards the floor to around chair height, then drive upwards in the same way you would if standing up from a chair. Repeat this movement. You can keep the chair in place if you feel more confident; just don't use it unless you have to!

Weighted squat: Start by standing with your feet shoulderwidth apart and your toes and eyes facing forwards. Select a weight or a household object and grip it with both hands, holding it at chest height, with your elbows tucked tightly to your sides. Now, keeping your back straight, bend your knees and allow your bum to lower to around chair height, before driving upwards with your bum and thigh muscles, until you are back to your starting position. Wearing a weighted rucksack also works very well for this movement. You can keep the chair in place if you feel more confident; just don't use it unless you have to!

For all versions of the squat, you should keep your back straight at all times.

Alternative – Wall sits (static): If you are unable to squat, try wall sits. Place your back flat against a wall and slowly allow your bum to slide towards the floor until your thighs are just above right angles – imagine you are sitting on a chair (you can place a chair, stool or sturdy box under you if this makes you feel more confident).

Start with 2 sets of 30 seconds, progressing to 2 sets of 2 minutes. Progress further to 3 sets of 2 minutes.

Also consider holding your weighted rucksack on your knees to increase the challenge of this movement.

You can progress in this movement by using a leg press machine or a bar-bell squat in a gym, with the advice of a qualified fitness professional.

7. Hip thrusts

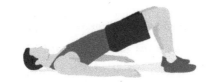

Hip thrust

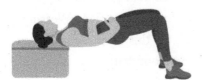 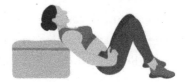

Body weight hip thrust

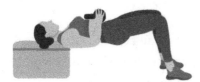 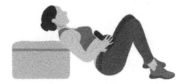

Weighted hip thrust

What?

This movement targets all the major muscles of the lower body but particularly the bum muscles (gluteals) and the back of the thighs (hamstrings). Think: standing up from a chair to an upright posture.

Why?

- Great for hip and lower-back strength and mobility
- Good for remaining independent, and getting on and off chairs and toilets unaided, and up from the floor
- Improves your ability to climb stairs in older age
- Improves your walking gait

- Protects your ability to stand up straight
- Stabilises the pelvis
- Works the largest muscles in the body
- Tones and shapes the bottom
- Maintains your ability to lift and carry everyday household items (or grandchildren!).

How?

Choose your starting point:

- Hip thrust
- Body weight hip thrust
- Weighted hip thrust (weights or household object needed)

Hip thrust: Lie on the floor, with your knees bent and your back and feet flat on the ground. Push your pelvis upwards with your weight carried between your shoulders and feet. The front of your thighs, pelvis and tummy should all be in line. Hold this for one second, then lower your bum back to the floor and repeat.

Body weight hip thrust: Start by resting your shoulders against a sofa, ensuring that your bum and feet are firmly planted on the floor and your knees are bent. Drive upwards in a thrusting movement with your hips so that the front of your thighs are in line with your abdomen and chest. Lower your bum back to the starting position.

Weighted hip thrust: Start by resting your shoulders against a sofa, ensuring that your bum and feet are firmly planted on the floor and your knees are bent. Place a weight or household object on your pelvis and hold it in place with both hands. Then drive upwards in a thrusting movement with your hips so that the front of your thighs are in line with your tummy and chest. Lower your bum back to the starting position. To progress from here, you can increase the weight that you use.

You can progress in this movement by using a hip thruster machine or exploring variations of the dead lift in a gym, with the advice of a qualified fitness professional.

8. Lunge

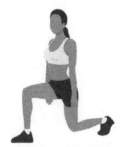

Body weight lunge

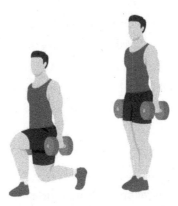

Weighted static lunge

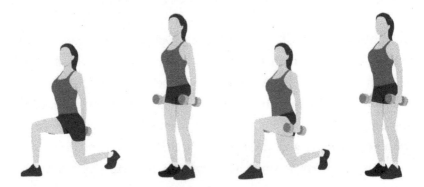

Weighted walking lunge

What?

This movement targets all the lower-limb muscles but primarily those in the front and rear of the thigh (quadriceps and hamstrings respectively) and the bum (gluteal). Think: picking something up from the floor.

Why?

- Great for general balance and lower-body strength
- An excellent all-round exercise for long-term hip, knee and ankle function and stability, which also protects against pain and injury
- Improves your ability to climb stairs in older age
- Improves your ability to get up from chairs or from sitting on the floor
- Improves your walking gait and reduces your risk of tripping
- Improves balance.

How?

Choose your starting point:
- Body weight lunge
- Weighted static lunge
- Weighted walking lunge

Body weight lunge: Start in the standing position, then step forwards with one foot as though you were taking a long step. Holding that position, with both feet facing forwards, allow your knees to bend. Lower your rear knee towards the ground, keeping your back straight and continuing to look forwards. Control the downward phase, stopping your rear knee a few inches from the floor. Then drive upwards with both legs to your starting position. Repeat this movement for the required number of reps on one side, then step back to the starting position with your feet together. Repeat this movement on the opposite side for the required number of reps. See *Foundation and Familiarisation phase* or *Next Steps* for guidance on numbers of sets and reps.

STRONGER

Weighted static lunge: Choose two identical household objects or weights and hold one in each hand. Let your arms fall to your sides, keeping them straight. Start in the standing position, then step forwards with one foot as though you were taking a long step. Holding that position, with both feet facing forwards, allow your knees to bend. Lower your rear knee towards the ground, keeping your back straight and continuing to look forwards. Control the downward phase, stopping your rear knee a few inches from the floor. Then drive upwards with both legs to your starting position. Repeat this movement for the required number of reps on one side, then step back to the starting position with your feet together. Repeat this movement on the opposite side for the required number of reps. Progress by holding heavier items or by wearing a weighted rucksack, taking care to keep your back straight. See *Foundation and Familiarisation phase* or *Next Steps* for guidance on numbers of sets and reps.

Walking lunge: I suggest starting with own bodyweight walking lunges for this version to familiarise yourself with the movement. Step forwards with one foot and allow your knees to bend. Lower your rear knee towards the ground with your front knee also bending whilst facing forwards. Keep your back straight and continue to look forwards. Control the downward phase, stopping your rear knee a few inches from the floor. Then drive upwards and step forwards with your opposite leg. Repeat the movement on alternate sides until you complete the required number of reps for both legs. Allow enough space and an even surface to perform this. You can then progress to the weighted version as you become more confident. (See *Foundation and Familiarisation phase* or *Next Steps*) for guidance on numbers of sets and reps.

Alternative – wall sits: If you find this movement, try wall sits (see page 132).

You can progress in this movement by using a sled push in a gym, with the advice of a qualified fitness professional.

Note: For all three of these movements, you can try the reverse lunge version, which involves stepping backwards instead of forwards (be careful not to trip over!).

9. Grip and lean, or grip and hang

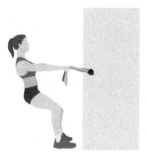

Grip and lean

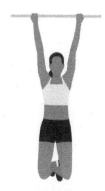

Grip and hang (pull-up bar required)

What?

This movement targets a wide range of muscles across the core, back and arms but in particular those we use to grip (the forearm and hands). Think: hanging from the monkey bars in a playground.

Why?

- Great all-round strengthening effect
- Improves your ability to save yourself from a trip or fall

- Ensures independence by improving your ability to grip everyday objects and tools
- Excellent for sports and recreational activities into older age
- Also good for shoulder stability, better sitting posture and protecting against neck pain.

How?

Choose your starting point:

- Grip and lean
- Grip and hang (requires pull-up bar).

Grip and lean: Secure a small towel by looping it around a banister or around door handles as shown in the image opposite. Facing the towel, grip it firmly with slightly bent knees and a straight back, leaning back slightly and allowing your elbows to straighten. Now hold this position statically – you should feel your body weight in your hands, forearms and shoulder blades. To progress, try placing your feet forwards and further away from you. You can place a chair just below your bum, so that if you need to rest or you lose your grip – you can just sit down!

Grip and hang: Grip the pull-up bar with your palms facing forwards and allow your body to hang whilst keeping as still as possible. Your feet should be off the floor and your arms fully straightened. If this is too challenging, you can place your feet on the floor to *unload* some of your body weight – hence decreasing the difficulty of gripping. You can gradually rely less on your feet as you progress. For even more progression, place a towel over the pull-up bar and grip it as you suspend your body weight below the pull-up bar as described.

Alternative – towel twist: Roll a hand towel until it matches your hand size. Grasp the towel with both hands, putting your arms out straight in front of you and squeezing tightly. Alternate rotating one wrist downwards and the other upwards to create a kind of wringing movement on the towel.

Start with 3 sets of 10 seconds, adding 2 seconds each time (see Chapter 6: *Minimal Loading Programme, towel twist*).

For all versions of this movement, aim to start with 2 sets of 15–30 seconds. Then build to 2 sets of 2 minutes before progressing by either changing the position of your feet (see: *grip and lean*) or trying more challenging versions of the movement (see: *grip and hang*).

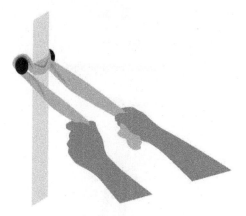

Securing your towel

10. Farmer's hold or walk

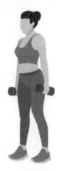

Farmer's hold (static)

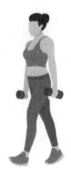

Farmer's walk

What?

This movement targets a wide range of muscles, including thighs, bottom, arms and back but in particular those we use to grip (the forearm and hands).

Why?

- Associated with greater longevity
- All-round strengthening effect
- Good for balance and leg, foot and ankle stability
- Improves your ability to save yourself from a trip or fall
- Ensures independence by improving your ability to grip tools, open things, carry shopping, household or garden items
- Improves your ability to carry heavy bags or luggage.

How?

Choose your starting point:

- Farmer's hold
- Farmer's walk.

Farmer's hold: Select two equal weights, or alternatively use two shopping bags or rucksacks weighed down with household objects, such as tins of food or water bottles or watering cans if outside. You will need to choose relatively heavy loads for this, otherwise it will be too easy. Standing still, keep your arms straight and by your sides whilst gripping a weight/object in each hand. Keep your back straight and core tight whilst breathing normally.

Aim to start with 2 sets of 30 seconds. To challenge yourself further, slowly increase your time and aim to get to 2 sets of 2 minutes before progressing to the walking version. You can make things more difficult by adding more objects to your bags or adding more water (if using watering cans). Once you can manage 2 sets of 2 minutes at a difficulty of 6–7 out of 10, you can progress to the farmer's walk.

Note: A 6–7 out of 10 difficulty equates to being able to grip for 2 sets of 2 minutes. Never go too far beyond your comfort zone so you drop things. When performing this movement, your sweet spot equates to holding for 2 minutes with the capacity to hold for another 20 seconds before you lose grip.

Farmer's walk: Choose your weights or objects as previously. With an upright posture, let your arms hang down straight by your sides. Hold one weight/object in each hand. Look straight ahead and make sure you have a clear route ahead of you. Gripping firmly on your weights/objects and keeping your core tight and your back straight, start to walk as normally as you can.

Note: Many people chose a circular route, meaning they start and finish at the same place. To progress with this movement, try adding load in the form of heavier weights. You can start at 2 sets of 30 seconds and build up to 2 sets of 2 minutes. From here further difficulty can be added by using a towel looped around the bag handle or weight, which you then grip and carry. You will probably need to decrease the weight used to accommodate the more challenging grip in the first instance.

Alternative: towel twist (see page 168)

Note: You should not push yourself to exhaustion or injury for any of these movements. Always strive to do quality training at a moderate to hard level whilst remaining in control. If you want to progress with your strength in ways other than described above, I urge you to seek coaching from a qualified fitness professional.

Using the Foundational 10 Movements

Here are the 3 phases to safely introduce long-term strength training into your life:

Phase 1: Preparation of your mind and body (this process started when reading this book!). This will take 2–4 weeks of the Minimal Loading Programme, see Chapter 6. Also see page 178 for *strength and balance snacking*.

Phase 2: Foundation and familiarisation to build functional muscle and strength and learn new movements whilst identifying your relative strengths and weakness. This will take 12 weeks (see below).

Phase 3: Maintain and develop your strength and power or train for a specific life goal. Ongoing for the rest of your life (see *Maintain and develop phase*, page 177, *FAQs*, page 182 and Next Steps, page 191).

Foundation and Familiarisation Phase

The initial Foundation and Familiarisation Phase lasts for 12 weeks in total. After this point, it can be repeated indefinitely in a cycle or alternated with other routines. In the first 8 weeks:

- Number of repetitions (reps): 10 (excluding grip or core, which are measured in length of time rather than reps)
- Number of sets: starting at 2
- Difficulty level: 6–7 out of 10 or moderately hard
- Perform each movement at constant speed, counting *one–two* on the way up and *one–two* on the way down (excluding grip and core exercises).

In the final 4 weeks:
- Add some *isometric* (static) contractions and some *eccentric* contractions (emphasis on longer lowering phases) into your training. Sometimes I keep things interesting in my own training by adding these elements into a single set of the given movement. For example, in a 10-rep set of press-ups, I would hold the press-up at halfway-up position for 2 seconds for the first 5 reps – and for the second 5 reps I would lower my chest slowly to the floor to the count of 4.

If you are feeling overly tired or sore, have a rest week and work on your flexibility. Also look to your sleep, rest, hydration and diet to see if anything can be improved.

Note: If you have completed the first 12-week Foundation and Familiarisation Phase and are thinking of using this framework as an indefinite rolling programme, you should include isometric and eccentric contractions within the programme from the beginning. See *FAQs* on page 188.

Aim to complete all Foundational 10 Movements twice a week (excluding core and grip exercises, which you only need to do once a week. This is due to their involvement in most of the other Foundational 10 Movements). However, when training grip, you can alternate between 9 and 10 each week, meaning that one week you can do the grip and lean movement and the next week you can do the farmer's hold movement.

How to progress

When 2 sets of 10 reps becomes easy, congratulate yourself. You have become stronger! Now increase to 3 sets of 10 and then 4 sets of 10, once 3 sets gets too easy.

Once you can perform 4 sets of 10 on your chosen starting point exercise, try to progress to a more difficult variation of the movement, initially dropping back down to 2 sets of 10 reps, before working up again towards 4 sets and 10 reps. If you have progressed to a more challenging version of a movement and 2 sets feels easy, add a third or fourth set until you feel you are at a 6–7 out of 10 level of challenge.

For progression in grip and core movements, we look at how long we can hold them, not how many times we do an individual rep. For both grip and core movements, start at 30 seconds and build to 2 minutes. Once you can hold for 2 minutes, add another set, starting at 30 seconds and building up again, until you are doing 2 sets of 2 minutes. You can add additional core sessions if you feel that one session of 2 x 2 minutes has become easy.

As mentioned earlier, you should aim to perform each movement in the Foundational 10 twice a week, excluding grip and core which can be trained once a week. If you're only able to incorporate the Foundational 10 once a week, you will still be building muscle and strength. Although twice is optimal, once is a whole lot better than nothing and any amount of training, if consistent over the long term, will go a long way. If you can train all movements at least once a week for the first 12 weeks, this is a great foundation. In time you will be able to add additional sessions – the most important thing is to make a start.

It is important to remember that the information shared within this book represents the current consensus on how often we need to train for muscle function and strength most effectively. The point here is that we just don't know what the perfect *dose* of strength training is for health in older age, which is why any amount of strength training, however small, has value. Everyone's needs will be different, and a single programme will never suit all of us.

A decade of competitive rowing has made me stronger at pulling than pushing in my upper body. However, a back injury means my lower-body strength does not match that of my upper body. Therefore, if I'm pushed for time, I prioritise lower-body and upper-body pushing movements, choosing to work on my relative areas of weakness. What are your strengths and weaknesses? Make sure you don't take the path of least resistance and prioritise the things you find easier! The real long-term health gold comes from working on our weaknesses.

Key points
- There is no right or wrong way. Find a weekly routine that suits your life at this time.
- Start with 2 sets of each movement and progress to 3 then 4 sets.
- Aim to train all movements (excluding core and grip) twice a week if possible.
- Your progression to more difficult movements or heavier weights may be different across the 10 movements and will be indicative of your stronger and weaker areas.
- If pushed for time, ensure you work on just those movements that you are not naturally strong in, returning to the full routine when you can.
- If you are not ready to start a regular structured programme, you might want to consider revisiting the *Minimal Loading Programme* we discussed in Chapter 6. This will go a long way towards protecting your joints and readying your body for when you can do more!
- Finally, I am a great believer in leveraging the activities of our everyday lives to improve our strength and balance. There is a great deal of benefit to be gained from just 5–10 minutes of strength activity a day, also known as 'strength snacking'. During lockdown, I became part of a working group called '10

today', which set out to develop quick, easy exercises for older people. During this time, I witnessed the cumulative benefits that even a few minutes of daily exercise can deliver if practised consistently over the long term. Subsequently, I have put together some suggestions for how to strength and balance snack (see page 178). Again, if this becomes your entry point into strength training, it will still count towards achieving the goals, which I earnestly hope you have started to write down on your strength bucket list.

Also see Next Steps: *How to plan your weekly routine* on page 193 for examples of how you could split the Foundational 10 Movements across a week.

Progression and plateaus

Although this plan may look arduous on paper, remember that for the purposes of our goal to 'finish strong' in older age, we need to frame our progress of strength through a longer-term lens.

We've all had experiences in exercise in which our fitness plateaus, and it's the same with strength training. No one can expect to increase and improve their strength indefinitely, because as we know, we lose muscle and strength as part of the ageing process. Therefore, at some point in the future, our strength progression will start to slow down. The point here is that, although we cannot avoid this happening completely, we will lose strength at a significantly slower rate than those who do not strength-train. With this in mind, a slower rate of loss can transform our ability to live the lives we want and achieve our strength goals.

A slower rate of strength loss still represents a huge win in the ageing game.

Pairing movements and 'super sets'

You will notice that I suggest pairing certain movements together (1 and 2, 3 and 4). This is because these paired movements use the opposite muscles to each other, which helps strengthen your body in a more balanced way. There is a great time-saving benefit to these 'super set' movements, in that you can transition straight from one to the other because they have not been fatigued by the work of their opposite number.

For example, if you were working on your upper body with a super set that combined a horizontal shoulder push with a horizontal shoulder pull, you could easily complete a set of press-ups then move straight to a set of exercise band pulls. Having completed both movements, you would then take your 2-minute rest before repeating or progressing to the next movement in that session.

To ensure you are working on the correct muscles for any of the 10 movements, look at the target muscle listed for each and if you are not feeling some tension or mild aching in that area, you should correct your form or technique until you do. If in doubt, seek advice from a qualified fitness professional.

Maintain and develop phase

Congratulations! Following the initial 12-week Foundation and Familiarisation Phase of training you will have built functional muscle, learned the movements, improved your strength and identified your relative strengths and weaknesses. It is now time to train for ongoing and long-lasting strength and power.

Your options now include the following:

- Exploring a change of focus to include more emphasis on strength and power by training at a *more challenging* level, with *fewer repetitions*. Or to put it another way: using the same Foundational 10 Movements, manipulating the difficulty level and rep range. For more on this, see Next Steps (page 191).
- Continuing to use the original Foundation and Familiarisation Phase as a rolling programme. Some of you might benefit from sticking to the original programme if you feel you are gaining and maintaining good levels of muscle and strength with this approach. (See FAQ on page 188: *Can I repeat the 12-week*

Foundation and Familiarisation Phase indefinitely?). This would mean using the original difficulty level and rep range and the including *all three contraction types* and *faster contractions for power*.

- Training specific movements for power/strength to improve a specific life activity or goal. This might be underpinning the strength required to continue or improve in a specific sport or hobby such as tennis, cycling or golf. Dr Tom Maden-Wilkinson, associate professor at the Advanced Wellbeing Research Centre at Sheffield Hallam University and co-founder of Strength for Life, suggested to me that a real-life goal can be a helpful motivation for strength training. He gave the example of an older gentleman whose main strength goal was to be able to continue to lift his grandchildren up. His strength training subsequently focused on building strength in the hip hinge movement and farmer's walk, enabling him to lift, hold and carry his grandchildren safely. Identify what your own goal may be and use it to identify which movements you want to focus on.

- Focusing your training to ensure you are enhancing your strength across all movements, paying particular attention to your weak spots.

- Exploring different approaches to developing your strength with a qualified personal trainer or strength and conditioning coach, and perhaps joining a gym.

- Harnessing everyday activities to get stronger and improve your balance!

Strength and balance snacking

Spread these strength and balance snacks across your normal working or home life. How many can you incorporate into your daily routine?

1. Stand on one leg whilst brushing your teeth or preparing food. This is great for both balance and strengthening the muscles of

your standing/weight-bearing side. Try brushing your teeth with the opposite hand whilst standing on one foot if safe to do so, to increase the challenge of balancing. The tiny adjustments your body makes in keeping you upright are gold dust for preventing trips and falls.

2. Try brushing your teeth whilst on tip-toes for sets of 10 seconds. This not only improves balance but also the strength of your legs, feet and toes. It's also great for foot mechanics and stability.

3. Consider being barefoot in the garden or around the house. This helps to naturally strengthen the small muscles of the foot, keeping arches healthy and improving stability.

4. Try 'doming' exercises for foot strength and mobility. To do this, take your shoes off, place a tissue or a pencil on the floor and attempt to pick it up using your toes. Do 3 sets of 10, alternating between feet. This can be done when relaxing at home in the evening or indeed under your work desk. Start with once a week, building to twice a week.

5. Hold an isometric (static) squat over the toilet for a short time or slowly lower your body weight onto the toilet seat (I have heard that some people hold this position when using a motorway service station toilet for reasons of hygiene, which I can fully understand!) Why not adopt this at work or indeed at home? It's a great way to work on the isometric strength of our thigh and bum muscles.

6. Keep a slight bend in your knees whilst prepping food. This slight bend is surprisingly effective at activating and strengthening the quadriceps muscle nearest the knee and is therefore great for our knee stability.

7. If you have a safe, quiet staircase (at work or home), try slowing your steps as you descend. Try counting *1-2-3* on each step down. Start with 5 steps for each leg and build up. (Do not try this in a busy stairwell!)

8. Use only three fingers whilst carrying shopping/a work bag or watering cans in the garden. This is a great way of turning grocery

shopping or gardening into an opportunity to build a stronger grip.

9. Stand up from seated at every opportunity possible. And when returning to the seated position, try pausing for a few seconds at the halfway down point. This is a great do-it-anywhere strengthening move for your hip and thigh muscles.

10. Always stand to put your socks on and avoid sitting to take them off. Not only is this a great workout in terms of balance, but it also requires you to contract the muscles in your standing leg and core in order to creates a stable stance. I practise this one every day because it means my foot, leg, thigh and hip muscles have to constantly adjust as I wrest that sock on. This is actually a very time-efficient and ageing-friendly habit that will protect us from falls in our older age.

11. Always take the stairs when there is a choice between stairs, lifts or escalators. Staircases are incredibly underrated opportunities for strengthing our lower bodies and maintaining balance. I always try to climb two at a time, if it's safe to do so. If your office has a staircase, try to find excuses to get out and about so you have no choice but to get those *stair reps* in.

12. When on the escalator of an underground system or shopping centre, always try to walk up and down, even if it is moving. Walking at pace on some escalators on the London underground actually represents a decent challenge – the Angel station underground escalator is the longest at just under 200ft – which can be good fun, especially if you have someone behind you who is in a hurry!

13. A great way of making the most of your rest and recovery between sets of training is what I call *garden and house reps*. Simply put, instead of sitting around waiting for 2 minutes between sets, you could do the recycling, empty the dishwasher, clean the kitchen, put a wash on etc. I have found that doing such tasks enables me to get my exercise and household duties ticked off at the same time. If training outside, I find a garden task to focus on between

sets, such as sweeping up leaves or pulling weeds. Far from being tiring, remaining gently active in our recovery periods can actually aid our muscles, getting us ready to train again more quickly. It also earns us domestic brownie points, so it's another midlife win-win!

14. I also try to control my breathing between sets of strength training (including if I am actively doing house or garden reps) via nose breathing. I particularly love to nose-breathe when taking my dog for a walk. This way of breathing is great for increasing our cardiovascular capacity without tiring us out. So the next time you are walking to work or around the supermarket, why not try it?

15. If you find yourself injured on one side of your body (e.g. your right shoulder), you can still offset some of the detraining on that joint by working on the other side (e.g. your left shoulder). For more on this, see Chapter 5: *Staying strong with an injury*. To minimise loss of strength and muscle mass it is important to keep strong in all uninjured areas if possible. You can do this by working on the lower body if the upper is injured and visa versa. If you find yourself immobilised due to injury or surgery, you may want to consider trying to contract your muscles without actually moving your joints, whilst obviously taking care not to aggravate your condition (for more on this see *Testing the connection* in Chapter 3). If all else fails and none of the above are feasible, I would still try to visualise myself strength-training every day because of the very real benefits this will confer to our nervous system. Given that research has shown that strength can return after detraining in the absence of increased muscle mass, we should respect the role of our nervous system in reacquiring strength after a long period of inactivity (for more on this see Chapter 3: *Watching and visualising exercise can get you stronger* and *A stronger sense of self and strengthening the brain*).

16. The final strength snack is for all those middle-aged males out there. If the thought of sitting to pee is anathema to you, I can relate, having held the same opinion until a few years ago.

However, my mind was changed in the course of my work and in observing the often-pivotal importance of being able to get on and off the toilet in terms of living independently. Bottom line – if you will pardon the pun – any middle-aged male who stands to pee is missing multiple opportunities a day to squat and in turn future-proof their ability to live independently.

If you have been injured and do not want to work at higher reps and moderately hard difficulty levels that's fine too. In fact, as we age, we can choose to work with the Foundational 10 Movements in whatever way suits our needs and supports our ability to keep turning up. Many older people gain a great deal of benefit from working at a lower-to-moderate difficulty level at higher rep ranges. You can still work on your strength when doing sets of 20 reps at 4–5 out of 10 level of difficulty.

Always keep in mind that higher rep numbers take longer, so are more likely to create discomfort in your muscles whilst you're training and an increased likelihood of delayed-onset muscle soreness (DOMS). See Chapter 5 for more on this.

Frequently asked questions (FAQs)

When do I start the Foundation and Familiarisation Phase?

Once you have completed the preparation phase (See Chapter 6: *Minimal Loading Programme* on page 126. If you are in good health and free from injury, you are ready to move on to the Foundation and Familiarisation Phase – see page 182: *The Foundational 10 Movements*.

How do I increase the difficulty of an exercise if my reps become too easy?

There are several ways of progressing as we get stronger, which include the following:

- Making the movement more difficult. For instance, in Movement 1, the horizontal shoulder push, you may start with a box press-up. As this becomes easier to do, gradually progress to doing a press-up. To progress from here, try a more difficult version of the press-up, such as a press-up with your feet on a chair, sofa or stair.
- If using weights, increasing the actual weight of the movement you work against.
- If using exercise bands, opting for a thicker one that offers more resistance.
- Varying the contraction type, such as adding eccentric or isometric movements. However, you should only do this after your first 8 weeks of training with the Foundation and Familiarisation Phase. See page 138: *The three types of muscle contraction* and page 173: *In the final 4 weeks*.
- Making grip movements harder by increasing the time you do an exercise for, or by increasing the difficulty of the grip (e.g. using a towel or alternating between selected fingers to grip for the farmer's hold/walk).
- Making core exercises harder by exploring different variations of the plank or increasing sets of transverse crunches.

How much rest do I need between sets of my workout?

Take 2 minutes minimum rest between different movements, unless you are combining movements (e.g. 1 and 2, 3 and 4) into super sets, in which case, rest after you have completed a paired set of movements. See: *Pairing movements and 'super sets'* on page 176. Make sure you are not feeling tired when starting a new set.

Do I need to do other exercise?
YES!

You may recall from Chapter 1 that good cardiovascular fitness decreases all-cause mortality dramatically, as does having good strength levels. A combination of the two will super-charge the odds of our last years being full and active. Remember when I mentioned we need to adopt a more hybrid approach to training? (See Chapter 6: *Hybrid workout*.)

Aim to train cardio at a level where you are not too out of breath to have a conversation (also known as 'Zone 2 training') at least 80-90% of the time and only push it harder (e.g. with interval training) for 10-20% of the time, depending on how much energy you have and how well you have slept. I was introduced to Zone 2 training as a method of increasing aerobic capacity or *base*, when I was a fire service physical training instructor. Walking briskly on an incline and jogging on flat ground or downhill is a tried and tested method, in both military and emergency services, of improving this capacity. Cycling, rowing machines, assault bikes and cross trainers are all also great ways of working on our Zone 2 for when we want to push things harder, as is any sport or activity that gets you slightly or more noticeably out of breath, such as gardening, brisk walking, cycling, tennis, football or swimming.

Try using some of the weekly splits to combine cardio and strength training. If you're doing them on the same day – which is perfectly fine for our purposes – train strength first and take care not to exhaust yourself I would suggest not training legs on the same day as cardio. You could also experiment with nose breathing during your Zone 2 training, as it's a great way of building greater respiratory capacity. Nose breathing increases the challenge of the activity without impacting our joints or inflicting excessive physical stress. (See page 178: *Strength and balance snacking*.)

Do I need equipment?

When starting out, most of the movements can be done without equipment. However, as you progress you might want to consider joining a gym or investing in some equipment. Exercise bands are relatively inexpensive, as are the majority of pull-up bars and exercise suspension systems. Adjustable dumb-bell sets also range from bespoke to inexpensive for those of us on a budget, as do home benches. (See Chapter 6: *Equipment list*.)

Is the programme the same when including eccentric or isometric elements?

Different contraction types can leave us feeling more fatigued. Therefore, be prepared to lower the challenge/weight of the movement in question and expect increased post-workout muscle soreness. You should also allow more recovery time between sets if you're feeling more fatigued.

Am I doing enough if I am only using body weight versions of the Foundational 10?

Yes, you are!

I would always encourage you to explore other ways of getting stronger, but rest assured – if you make it to elevated feet press-ups, unassisted pull-ups, walking lunges, 2 minutes of plank and farmer's walk, by anyone's definition, you will be strong! The goal is to progress as far as you can and then hold that level for as long as you can.

Should I do anything different in relation to the menopause?

I would strongly recommend strength training during this time as lower oestrogen levels often have a negative impact on bone health. Strength training maintains muscle, which as we know, will protect us from osteoporosis. Additionally, specialised cells within our bones sense the mechanical forces we expose our skeleton to during strength training and they respond by laying down thicker and stronger bone. So, it turns out that strength training is one of the most effective things we can do in the prevention of osteoporosis. A body-wide programme, strengthening all major muscle groups – like the *Foundational 10* – will also protect all our bones. For more on this revisit Chapter 1.

Should I do anything different around my monthly period?

How you feel should dictate if or how hard you train. If you do strength-

STRONGER

train, ensure your protein intake is around 1.5g per kg of body weight per day as a minimum. For more on this, See Chapter 1: *Diet and digestion* (page 28).

Can I do more than the Foundational 10 Movements recommended?

The Foundational 10 is specifically aimed at middle-aged people wanting to learn how to strength-train. The volume of training suggested is also designed to avoid fatigue or injury from over training. You can do more, but just listen to your body and keep track of how you feel or are performing. Also see Next Steps (page 191).

What if I can't do a particular movement from the Foundational 10?

Many of us have old or existing injuries that may stop us from doing some of the Foundational 10 – and that is fine. Whatever your injury or condition, there is usually a way to train that does not aggravate things. Perhaps have a look at Chapter 5 or seek the advice of a qualified health or fitness professional for alternative ways of strengthening a particular movement. Remember that the static exercises in the Minimal Loading Programme will do a good deal to preserve our long-term strength (see Chapter 6: *Minimal Loading Programme*).

How can I work on my balance?

Almost any daily activity or exercise can be adapted to include an element of balance. I try to train this every day, if only for a few minutes. Most of the Foundational 10 Movements can be adapted for more focus on balance. For example, Movement 3 (vertical shoulder push) can include going onto your tiptoes at the top of the push. Movement 8 (walking lunge) and Movement 10 (farmer's walk) are also great for balance. Also see page 178: *Strength and balance snacking*.

Is there anything I can do to get stronger when my work is sedentary?

Just like balance, almost any daily activity can be adapted to elicit strength benefits (see page 178: *Strength and balance snacking*).

How should I structure my workout?

The six gears of any workout should include the following:

- Thinking about the exercise you are about to do, thereby prepping your nervous system.
- Warming up the body, thereby activating the mind–body connection. This can be any activity that gets you moving and brings a slight increase in heart rate (5–10 minutes of a gentle exercise such as a brisk walk around the block whilst swinging your arms back and forth).
- Completing the required sets with emphasis on the quality of your form.
- Warming down and stretching to return your body to normal.
- Breathwork (or other calming techniques), which enable your nervous system to get into a parasympathetic state more quickly. (See Chapters 3 and 4 for why this helps our long-term strength.)
- Celebrating your effort and the fact that you are building a future that is stronger.

What should I do if I my strength is not progressing?

In the initial 12 weeks of the Foundational 10 programme, you are likely to progress in all target areas. If, however, you find yourself not progressing, be sure to check your diet, rest, hydration and other life pressures that might be affecting your training and recovery. Remember that progress will be different across the 10 movements and for different people.

What if I am pushed for time and have to choose between cardiovascular and strength training?

This is a question that comes up a great deal with middle-aged people. So much so that I put this very question to one of the most knowledgeable physical activity experts in the UK. Professor Greg Whyte OBE is a former British Olympic pentathlete, still competing in ultra-endurance events at an elite level, and an authority in exercise physiology, sports performance and rehabilitation. 'If I had to choose, it would without doubt be strength training, because of the many protective benefits that we know it delivers for ageing.'

Hopefully none of us will ever be that busy, or think we are so busy, that such a decision has to be made. That said, on occasions when our diaries do curtail our normal training routines, I would endeavour to find the time to maintain my strength, given the rapidity at which we can lose this most precious of health assets. To address this issue, in addition to the Foundational 10 Movements, I have compiled a list of opportunities we can integrate into our everyday lives to get stronger – see page 178: *Strength and balance snacking*.

Can I repeat the 12-week Foundation and Familiarisation Phase indefinitely?

The short answer is yes – but with a caveat. I would always suggest some variation within your training programme, such as including all three contraction types (see page 138: *The three types of muscle contraction*) and faster contractions that promote more power. (See the next FAQ; and Next Steps on page 191 for more on this.)

If you are using this programme in the long term, be sure to incorporate the different contraction types and power work from Week 1. This might look like performing your first set with more speed and then including isometric or eccentric elements in the other sets.

Having a defined break at the end of any period of training is also a great way to recover fully and avoid overtraining. A one- or two-week pause is therefore a good idea at the end of the 12 weeks, but only if you include other activities in your life that are challenging in different ways from strength training. For example, tennis, badminton, skipping, climbing, sprints, fast walking, hiking with a weighted rucksack will all activate those all-important fast-twitch fibres that you've gone to the trouble of training because once we have them, we should endeavour to keep them working well!

If you need to take a longer break from your training, try to find ways of actively using these fibres (see page 178: *Strength and balance snacking*).

After your initial 12-week Foundation and Familiarisation Phase, it really is up to you to decide how you want to continue. Many participants benefit from alternating between the exercises in the Foundation and Familiarisation Phase and working with the same movements, albeit at a more challenging difficulty level, and lower reps as described in the *Maintain and develop phase* on page 177).

I personally like to alternate between these two programmes every six weeks with a short break between for a nice variation and to keep things interesting. This way I get 6 weeks of training focused on building functional muscle and strength (using the difficulty level, sets and rep range from the Foundation and Familiarisation Phase, followed by 6 weeks of training with more emphasis on increasing strength and power (using the difficulty level, set and rep range from the Next Steps programme on page 191).

Are there other ways to improve or maintain power?

You may recall from Chapter 1 and 3 that faster movements help us preserve our all-important fast-twitch fibres , as well as the ability of our nervous system to control them. This is significant because it is this relationship – between muscle and nervous system – that dictates our strength, power and health in older age.

Broadly speaking, there are two ways we can work on power, both requiring the application of more speed. Firstly, using the Foundational Movements (excluding grip and core), we can attempt to conduct the movement more rapidly than we have previously.

Secondly, we can utilise other methods to generate more powerful muscle contractions. Look at slam balls (robust semi-solid balls that can be lifted, thrown or slammed down and dropped without damage), or plyometrics (for example, jumping up onto an exercise box and stepping off). Also look at skipping, throwing, punch-bag boxing drills, short all-out sprints and basically anything involving short, sharp spells of physical activity, allowing full recovery between efforts.

Any sport or activity involving throwing a ball or swinging a bat, club or racket are all great for power. In fact, any movement completed as fast as possible, whilst under some kind of load, will improve our ability to quickly generate power.

Note: 5–10 minutes of skipping is great for your warm-up and targets your fast-twitch fibres.

Next Steps

You now have the option to change the way you use the Foundational 10 Movements to train for strength and power.

How

1. Increase the difficulty of the movements
Also see FAQ: *How do I increase the difficulty of an exercise?*

Number of reps = 5.
5 reps at a more challenging level brings optimal strength gains.

This means you will choose your starting point based on your ability to perform 5 reps.

You should be feeling like the fifth rep is challenging, but you are in control. Remember, if you can't complete the fifth rep you are working too hard.

Number of sets = starting at 2 and rising to 4.
When 2 sets of 5 reps becomes easy, increase to 3 sets of 5 and then 4 sets of 5, once 3 sets gets too easy. Once you can perform 4 sets of 5 on your chosen starting point exercise, try to progress to a more difficult variation of the movement, initially dropping back down to 2 sets of 5 reps, before working up again towards 4 sets and 5 reps.

Note: If you have progressed to a more challenging version of a movement and 2 sets feels easy, add a third or fourth set until you feel you are at an 8 out of 10 level of challenge.

Difficulty level = feels more like an 8 out of 10 effort.
This should feel more challenging than the Foundation and Familiarisation Phase.

You should be capable of 5 reps, with the ability to do another 2 reps before having to stop, i.e. you have 2 reps in reserve, which you do not use.

Core and grip movements = remain unchanged from Foundation and Familiarisation Phase.

1) Train for more power using faster contractions with emphasis on increased speed. This would mean a faster upward phase of a movement, such as a press-up, lunge or squat, or increasing the speed of the pulling phase of a pull-up or banded pull. If doing 4 sets of a movement, I like to do the first set for power then revert to the standard speed in the other sets.

   Note: Reps remain at 5 when working on power in the Next Steps programme.

   Reps remain at 10 when working on power in the Foundation and Familiarisation phase. See: FAQ – *Can I repeat the 12 week Foundation and familiarisation phase indefinately?*.

2) Include variations of all three contraction types (see page 138). I might choose to include isometric and eccentric contractions during one of my sets. For the vertical shoulder push, this would look like a 1–2-second pause at the halfway point up or down for isometric and a longer 4-second lowering phase in the eccentric rep. Alternatively, one week I might choose to work only on isometric or eccentric for one set. The point here is that it's OK to try out different things.

3) Increase the number of sets you are doing. This might mean increasing the total number of sets of each movement to 10 per week (excluding grip and core).

Why

Increasing the difficulty of an exercise develops and maintains our neuromuscular ability to contract the muscle (See Chapter 3 for why this is important for preserving strength).

Training for power helps preserve our fast-twitch fibres into older age (see Chapters 1 and 3 for why this is should be a priority).

Variation in contraction types or weekly routines is great for continuing gains in functional muscle and strength. Remember, such variations will keep our bodies *guessing and progressing*, helping us preserve our strength and power.

Increasing the volume of weekly sets ensures continued progression of strength and power.

How to plan your weekly routine

Below are some examples of how to organise your training across a week.

The suggested weekly splits below remain the same for both the Foundation and Familiarisation Phase and the Next Steps Programme – albeit with differences in the level of difficulty and rep ranges.

2 sessions per week

Start with 2 sets of each movement – rising to 4 sets.

Monday: Full body and core.

Tuesday: Rest.

Wednesday: Rest.

Thursday: Full body and grip.

Friday: Rest.

Saturday: Rest.

Sunday: Rest

The 2-day strength plan would flow something like this:

Full body

Movement 1 then 2 (horizontal shoulder push then horizontal shoulder pull). Rest and then repeat, or move to next movement once you have completed the required sets.

Movement 3 then 4 (vertical shoulder push then vertical shoulder pull). Rest and repeat or move to next movement.

Core and grip

Movement 6 then 7 then 8 (squat and rest, hip thrust and rest, lunge and rest). Repeat or move to next movement.

As you are training all movements twice over 2 separate days, you can either choose to include Movement 5 (plank) or Movements 9 or 10 (grip) on the days you are working your full body or on other days across the week.

6 sessions per week

Start with 2 sets of each movement – rising to 4 sets. Make sure you have a rest between each movement.

Monday: Working your upper body (horizontal movements).
- Horizontal shoulder push (1) and horizontal shoulder pull (2).
- 10–20 mins.

Tuesday: Working your lower body.
- Squat (6), hip thrust (7) and lunge (8), then plank (5).
- 10–30 mins.

Wednesday: Working your upper body (vertical movements).
- Vertical shoulder push (3) and vertical shoulder pull (4).
- 10–20 mins.

Thursday: Working your upper body (horizontal movements).
- Horizontal shoulder push (1) and horizontal shoulder pull (2).
- 10–20 mins.

Friday: Working your lower body.
- Squat (6), hip thrust (7) and lunge (8), then grip and lean or grip and hang (9) or farmer's hold or walk (10).
- 10–30 mins.

Saturday: Working your upper body (vertical movements).
- Vertical shoulder push (3) and vertical shoulder pull (4).
- 10–20 mins.

Sunday: Rest.

Note: You could train core and grip movements (5 or 9 and 10) on Sundays or train them on different days across the week.

Alternative

Some people split their training week into upper- and lower-body days:

Monday: Upper-body movements (1, 2, 3, 4)
Tuesday: Lower-body movements (6, 7, 8)
Wednesday: Core and grip movements (5, 9, 10)
Thursday: Upper-body movements (1, 2, 3, 4)
Friday: Lower-body movements (6, 7, 8)
Saturday and Sunday: Rest.

The sessions would flow something like this:

Upper body

Movements 1 and 2 (Horizontal shoulder push and horizontal shoulder pull), rest and then repeat, until you complete the required sets.

Movements 3 and 4 (Vertical shoulder push and vertical shoulder pull), rest and repeat until you complete the required sets.

Lower body

Movements 6, 7, 8 (squat and rest, hip thrust and rest, lunge and rest), then repeat until you complete the required sets.

Core and grip

Plank and rest, then grip and lean or farmer's hold, rest and repeat until you complete the required sets.

Endnotes

Introduction

1. Li R, Xia J, Zhang XI, Gathirua-Mwangi WG, Guo J, Li Y, McKenzie S, Song Y. Associations of Muscle Mass and Strength with All-Cause Mortality among US Older Adults. *Med Sci Sports Exerc*. 2018 Mar;50(3):458-467. doi: 10.1249/MSS.0000000000001448. PMID: 28991040; PMCID: PMC5820209.

2. Rosenberg, H. Sarcopenia: origins and clinical relevance. *The Journal of nutrition* 127.5 (1997): 990S-991S.

3. UK Active. 2017. www.ukactive.com/events/inactive-brits-spend-twice-as-long-on-toilet-per-week-as-they-do-exercising/

4. Sandercock GRH, Moran J, Cohen DD. Who is meeting the strengthening physical activity guidelines by definition: A cross-sectional study of 253 423 English adults? *PLoS One*. 2022 May 4;17(5):e0267277.

5. Public Health England. Adult and older persons Physical Activity Guide. www.gov.uk/government/publications/physical-activity-guidelines-adults-and-older-adults; World Health Organization. Physical Activity. https://www.who.int/initiatives/behealthy/physical-activity#:~:text=For%20additional%20health%20benefits%2C%20adults,or%20more%20days%20a%20week

6. Cooper R, Gita G, Mishra D, Kuh D. Physical activity across adulthood and physical performance in Midlife. Findings from a British Birth cohort. *American Journal of Preventative Medicine*. 2011;41(4) 376-384.

7. Skelton DA, Mavroeidi A. How do muscle and bone strengthening and balance activities (MBSBA) vary across the life course, and are there particular ages where MBSBA are most important? J *Frailty, Sarcopenia and Falls*. 2018 Jun 1;3(2):74-84. doi: 10.22540/JFSF-03-074. PMID: 32300696; PMCID: PMC7155320.

8. Araujo CG, de Souza e Silva CG, Laukkanen JA, et al. Successful 10-second one-legged stance performance predicts survival in middle-aged and older individuals. *British Journal of Sports Medicine* 2022;56:975-980.

9. Increasing life expectancy. www.macrotrends.net/countries/GBR/united-kingdom/life-expectancy

Chapter 1

1. Wall BT, Gorissen SH, Pennings B, Koopman R, Groen BBL, et al. (2015) Aging Is Accompanied by a Blunted Muscle Protein Synthetic Response to Protein Ingestion. *PLOS ONE* 10(11): e0140903.

2. Morton RW, Murphy KT, McKellar SR, et al. A systematic review, meta-analysis and meta-regression of the effect of protein supplementation on resistance training-induced gains in muscle mass and strength in healthy adults. *British Journal of Sports Medicine* 2018;52:376-384.

3. Guasch-Ferré, M, Willett, WC. The Mediterranean diet and health: a comprehensive overview. *Journal of Internal Medicine* 2021; 290: 549–566.

4. Kim CH, Wheatley CM, Behnia M, Johnson BD. The Effect of Aging on Relationships between Lean Body Mass and VO2max in Rowers. *PLOS ONE.* 2016;11(8):e0160275. Published 2016 Aug 1. doi:10.1371/journal. pone.0160275

5. Volpi E, Nazemi R, Fujita S. Muscle tissue changes with ageing. *Current Opinion in Clinical Nutrition and Metababolic Care.* 2004 Jul;7(4):405-10. doi: 10.1097/01.mco.0000134362.76653.b2. PMID: 15192443; PMCID: PMC2804956.

6. Tian Y, Thompson J, Buck D, Sonola L. Exploring the system-wide costs of falls in older people in Torbay. *The Kings Fund.* 2013. kingsfund.org.uk.

7. Kevin Fenton. The Human Cost of Falls. 2014. UK Health Security Agency. https://ukhsa.blog.gov.uk/2014/07/17/the-human-cost-of-falls/

8. Kevin Fenton. The Human Cost of Falls. 2014. UK Health Security Agency. https://ukhsa.blog.gov.uk/2014/07/17/the-human-cost-of-falls/

9. Burns E, Kakara R. Deaths from Falls Among Persons Aged ≥65 Years - United States, 2007-2016. *The Morbidity and Mortality Weekly Report.* 2018;67(18):509-514. Published 2018 May 11. doi:10.15585/mmwr. mm6718a1.

10. Rogeri PS, Gasparini SO, Martins GL, et al. Crosstalk Between Skeletal Muscle and Immune System: Which Roles Do IL-6 and Glutamine Play?. *Front Physiol.* 2020;11:582258. Published 2020 Oct 16. doi:10.3389/fphys.2020.582258

11. Nelke, C et al. Skeletal muscle as a potential central link between sarcopenia and immune senescence. *eBioMedicine.* 2019; 49, P381-388.

Chapter 3

1. Plotkin DL, Roberts MD, Haun CT, Schoenfeld BJ. Muscle Fiber Type Transitions with Exercise Training: Shifting Perspectives. *Sports (Basel).*

2021;9(9):127. Published 2021 Sep 10. doi:10.3390/sports909012

2. Miljkovic N, Lim JY, Miljkovic I, Frontera WR. Ageing of skeletal muscle fibers. *Annals of Rehabilitation Medicine.* 2015 Apr;39(2):155-62. doi: 10.5535/arm.2015.39.2.155. Epub 2015 Apr 24. PMID: 25932410; PMCID: PMC4414960.

3. Andersen JL, Klitgaard H, Saltin B. Myosin heavy chain isoforms in single fibres from m. vastus lateralis of sprinters: influence of training. *Acta Physiologica Scandinavica* 151.2 (1994): 135-142.

4. Behm DG, Sale DG. Intended rather than actual movement velocity determines velocity-specific training response. *Journal of Applied Physiology* 74.1 (1993): 359-368.

5. Alan Turing Institute. Data Study Group Final Report: eGym Improved strength training using smart gym equipment data. 2018.

6. Taaffe DR, Marcus R. Dynamic muscle strength alterations to detraining and retraining in elderly men. *Clinical Physiology and Functional Imaging.* 1997 May;17(3):311-24. doi: 10.1111/j.1365-2281.1997.tb00010.x. PMID: 9171971.

7. Abe T, Loenneke JP, Thiebaud RS, Fukunaga T. Age-related site-specific muscle wasting of upper and lower extremities and trunk in Japanese men and women. *Age (Dordr).* 2014 Apr;36(2):813-21. doi: 10.1007/s11357-013-9600-5. Epub 2013 Nov 17. PMID: 24243442; PMCID: PMC4039273.

8. Coyle, Daniel. *The Talent Code.* Arrow Books. 2010.

9. Buccino, G. Action observation treatment: a novel tool in neurorehabilitation, *Philosophical Transactions of the Royal Society B.* 2014 Jun 5; 369(1644): 20130185.

10. Robinson, David. *The Expectation Effect.* Canongate Books. 2022.

11. Sir Charles Sherrington – Facts. NobelPrize.org. Nobel Prize Outreach AB 2022. Mon. 21 Nov 2022. <https://www.nobelprize.org/prizes/medicine/1932/sherrington/facts.

Chapter 4

1. Radvansky G, Tamplin AK, and Kraweitz SA, Walking Through Doorways Causes Forgetting: Environmental Integration. *Psychonomic Bulletin and Review,* 2010 Dec. 17(6):900-4. doi: 10.3758/PBR.17.6.900.

2. Sinclair, Dr David. *LifeSpan.* Atrial Books. 2019.

3. The next era of Human-Machine Partnerships. Emerging Technologies Impact on Society and Work in 2030. Institute for the Future and Dell technologies. 2017.

4. Sanfilippo, Lisa. *Yoga Therapy for Insomnia and Sleep Recovery*. Singing Dragon Books. 2019.

5. Cohen-Hatton SR, Butler PC, Honey RC. An Investigation of Operational Decision Making in Situ: Incident Command in the U.K. Fire and Rescue Service. *Human Factors*. 2015 Aug;57(5):793-804. doi: 10.1177/0018720815578266. Epub 2015 Mar 30. PMID: 25875155.

6. Sechenov, Ivan. *Reflexes of the Brain*. 1863. Translated by MIT Press. 1965.

7. Cooper R, Strand B H, Hardy R, Patel K V, Kuh D. Physical capability in mid-life and survival over 13 years of follow-up: British birth cohort study *British Medical Journal* 2014; 348 :g2219 doi:10.1136/bmj.g2219.

8–10. Glover IS, Baker SN. Cortical, Corticospinal and Reticulospinal Contributions to Strength Training. *Journal of Neuroscience*. 22 July 2020.

11. Robinson, David. *The Expectation Effect*. Canongate Books. 2022.

Chapter 5

1. FA Worsley. Superhuman effort isn't worth a damn unless it achieves results. In: *Endurance*. WW Norton and Company. 1999.

2. Fayaz A, Croft P, Langford RM, Donaldson LJ, Jones GT. Prevalence of chronic pain in the UK: a systematic review and meta-analysis of population studies. *British Medical Journal* Open. 2016 Jun 20;6(6):e010364. doi: 10.1136/bmjopen-2015-010364. PMID: 27324708; PMCID: PMC4932255.

3. Moseley GL, Butler DS, 15 Years of Explaining Pain – The Past, Present and Future. *Journal of Pain* 2015;10:1016

4. Melzack R, Wall PD. Pain mechanisms: a new theory. *Science*. 1965 Nov 19;150(3699):971-9

5. Pleger B, et al. Repetitive transcranial magnetic stimulation induced changes in sensorimotor coupling parallel improvements of somatosensation in humans. *Journal of Neuroscience*. 2006; 26: 1945–1952.

6. Wallden M. Rehabilitation and movement re-education. In: Chaitow L (Ed.). *Naturopathic Physical Medicine*. London: Churchill Livingstone, 2008.

7. Sinclair, Dr David. *LifeSpan*. Atrial Books. 2019.

Chapter 6

1. Okun MS, Mayberg HS, DeLong MR. Muhammad Ali and Young-Onset Idiopathic Parkinson Disease—The Missing Evidence. *JAMA Neurology*. 2023;80(1):5–6. doi:10.1001/jamaneurol.2022.3584

Index

Author biography

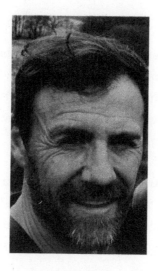

David Vaux is recognised as one of the UK's most innovative osteopaths, with a special interest in strength and movement prescription for optimal ageing and pain management.

He began his career working as a London firefighter, serving for 15 years on fire rescue operations and as physical education officer until he suffered a career-ending injury. He subsequently retrained as an osteopath, applying strength and movement research to his own rehabilitation whilst gaining two master's degrees in the process.

David uses his lived and clinical experience to provide injury-reducing conditioning advice within performing arts and international sports. In addition to this, he provides strategic advice on exercise to UK charities, think tanks and healthy-ageing steering groups. He is an authority on older-age strength and resilience, and over the last decade has advised on projects feeding into the UK Government's Ageing Society Grand Challenge.

David's new rescue mission is the democratisation of strength for all, in the fight for optimal immunity, independent ageing and resilience.

Acknowledgements

I am immensely grateful for the time that has been given to me when researching this book. In particular, Mr Martin Lau, Professor Rachel Cooper, Professor Greg Whyte OBE and Professor Tom Maden-Wilkinson for sharing their insights and experiences when working to help people live better for longer.

Thanks also to my friend James Blanchard and James Geering for planting the seed of this book in my mind and my other friends for their endless positivity. To my Fire Brigade brothers, Mike and Nam, thank you for showing me the true meaning of support and friendship.

Tom Drake Lee was instrumental in helping me find my voice as a writer and opening the door into the literary world. I am grateful for his professionalism and boundless encouragement in the early days of this project.

I owe a debt of gratitude to my agent Jane for believing in this book and to Amy for her tireless support, whilst also allowing me to keep (if only a few of) the puns! I also need to acknowledge the opportunity that was given to me by Octopus Books and my editor Helena for immediately understanding my vision whilst carefully guiding my concept into reality.

I also want to acknowledge my family and the countless inspirational people that have enriched my life with their wisdom. Finally, I would like to thank my fiancée Sarah for her love and support, without which I would not have been strong enough to complete this challenge.